Another Name for Madness

Another Name for Madness

Marion Roach

Houghton Mifflin Company

Boston   1985

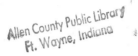
Library of Congress Cataloging in Publication Data

Roach, Marion.
Another name for madness.

1. Roach, Allene, 1928–   2. Alzheimer's
disease—Patients—United States—Biography.   I. Title.
RC523.R63R63   1985   618.97′683 [B]   85-4297
ISBN 0-395-35373-4

Printed in the United States of America

S 10 9 8 7 6 5 4 3 2 1

To my family —

my mother, my father, and my sister

Another Name for Madness

Chapter 1

I ALWAYS SAY that it started when my mother killed the cats. She took four of her seven precious felines to the vet and had them destroyed. I wanted to believe she had momentarily gone mad. But the thought didn't last long.

The cats trusted her. Five of them slept around her every night. The other two found other spots; their favorite, where they lay curled together, was among the hammers in the baby grand piano when the top was left open. Every morning, in the kitchen, the seven cats would swirl around my mother's ankles at the first stir of the day. In those days my mother always got up early. Her favorite expression was "Be up. Be doing." She was always up — and doing something — by six.

One October morning, my mother grabbed two cats by the shoulders and carried out one in each fist — limp purses swinging in her grasp — and tossed them into the car. I followed her, at first just watching. She didn't flinch as their paws slid across the seat. I don't think she noticed that their legs splayed like dropped pick-up sticks and that their fur retained a deep imprint from her large palms.

I noticed.

The cats seemed to think that being thrown in the car was

a game. The window on the driver's side was down, and the two cats hit the seat, then leaped out to the street, trotted around the car, and sat — grooming, licking paws — on the grass. My mother rolled up the window, picked up one cat and then the other, hurled them back into the car, and slammed the door.

She marched back into the house and got another cat. As its legs collapsed on the seat, I thought of the time my father's friend Pat sat in my baby chair when I was a child. Its legs went out at four angles. I stood there, looking through the window at the cats, and thought of Pat, spilling his drink. I couldn't accept that my mother was really doing this. Finally, I had to.

"Mommy," I cried, sounding more like a child than a woman of twenty-three, "what are you doing? Have you gone mad?"

"No, dammit," she said. "I don't want to feed them any-more. I don't and I won't. I don't want to feed them anymore."

She had her teeth clenched and was speaking through them, looking straight ahead at nothing.

Eva, the housekeeper, wept. I tried to, but I kept watching my mother. She returned to the house and found one more cat downstairs in the hall, where she had collected the seven. The others seemed to be trying to avoid her. My mother had become a machine, picking up and hurling cats and churning out the same words.

I tried to reason with her. "Mommy, come on, the cats haven't done anything. Let's keep them."

"No," she said firmly.

As always, she had the final say. She was my mother. It was her house.

No boxes, no restraints; the cats sat in the car; a tableau that remains searingly clear to this day, a flash bulb after-image I would like to forget.

My mother drove with the cats to the vet and returned with a handful of collars and a receipt. She had had the cats injected with something to put them to sleep.

She got four.

The thought that my mother was losing her mind lasted exactly as long as it took me to ask her if she was crazy and for her to answer no. From that moment on, as she silently fought an illness that was stealing her awareness, I welcomed a denial that stole mine: she couldn't be going mad. Not her.

My sister, Margaret, doesn't deny. She confronts. Margaret, who is two years older than I, lived in California at the time my mother took the cats to be destroyed. It was the fall of 1979, and our father had been dead for a year and a half. My mother and I lived together.

I telephoned Margaret to tell her about the cats. There was a pause on the phone before Margaret asked me to repeat the story. She asked me how I felt about it. It seemed an irrelevant question. She said that it wasn't. My sister insisted that I take my mother to a neurologist. She also said that that there had been something wrong with our mother for over a year.

"Come on, Marion," she said; "losing her keys, coming home late. What about her coat?"

I had told Margaret the week before that our mother had stopped talking about having her fur coat shortened. Until then, it had been a preoccupation. The coat was much longer than was the fashion at the time, and she had been obsessed by it — talking about it over and over — and then she just dropped the subject. My mother also ate yogurt every night for dinner. She had stopped cooking.

"Marion, don't you think all these things add up to something?"

"No."

. . .

Three weeks later, in the middle of November, my mother and I are sitting in the waiting room of a neurologist's office.

My sister has prevailed.

My mother is so beautiful that I dress up even to take her to the doctor. I am fidgeting with my skirt when the doctor calls us in.

As he asks her name and address, I sit looking out the window, down First Avenue. I wonder what the people in the cars are thinking about, staring at their windshields. My mother is sitting in a chair, holding on to her seat, her long nails scraping at the underside of the wide leather sling. The sound of her nails on the rough suede is what wrenches me from my daydream.

"Mrs. Roach, what is the date?" asks the doctor.

"May," she blurts out.

May? I feel an odd horror. It's cold outside. May, I repeat to myself. How can she think it's May?

During the next hour she correctly subtracts by sevens from one hundred, draws pictures, is told to remember three words, is asked them a few minutes later, and can't remember them.

We go through her life history, starting with the present and working back, and the farther back we get, the more she remembers. Yesterday is a blank, and the week before. She knows that she worked as a teacher for nearly ten years; she gives the address of the school and the name of her assistant.

"Is this correct?" asks the doctor of me, as he does after each of her answers. He is asking me to say, in front of her, "No, we no longer have seven cats; we have three," and "Yes, we live in the town in which she grew up," and "Those are the right names of the witnesses at her wedding." As the questions get farther and farther away from the present, and farther in time from the ones she answered incorrectly, they become easier for her to embroider with correct details, and she smiles and relaxes. So do I, and things seem just fine.

"Mrs. Roach, when were you born?"

"November 6, 1928. My mother was out planting tulips and never got to vote for Herbert Hoover."

"Is this correct?" he asks me.

"Yes," I say, smiling at my mother. It's one of our favorite stories.

Chapter 2

MY GRANDMOTHER, Marion Rollins Zillmann, was outside planting tulips when she got the first pain. It was November 6, 1928, and even though there was the first snap of winter, she was still in her garden.

Before she married, Marion Rollins had been one of those dark-eyed girls with piled-up hair who are now famous in old posters. She was also one of the young women in Wisconsin who received a telegram in 1918 telling her that her fiancé had been killed in France.

Before that, she had been in high school and in love with Fredric March (and he, she said, with her) when he was still Frederick McIntyre Bickel from Racine, Wisconsin. She knew she had done the right thing, staying home and marrying a handsome young man just back from the war instead of following a man and his dream of being an actor to New York, but as she read and reread the telegram through the years, she wondered if she'd made the right choice.

When she first received the telegram, people told her the right thing to do was to keep busy. But they didn't have to tell her that. Marion had already begun the process of rereading and numbering the letters from France. She stacked the sheets with the large American eagle watermark on her desk. He had written of the trenches "three feet deep with a little piece of tin over me for shelter from the big shells that fall all the time. A person couldn't even stick his head above ground during daylight, which means that we lay in bed for sixteen hours a day." He went on to tell of a mess crew working its way through the tent with a huge vat of stew, a barrel of coffee, and a platter of sandwiches during a shell strike and of one officer's diving into the stew. He wrote to her to tell "anyone who has designs on you that I'll be back soon."

That letter arrived two weeks after the telegram. Grandma Zillmann was practical, even with her emotions. She numbered that last letter 130 and drew a circle around the number.

Several other luckier young soldiers had indeed had designs on her before the war changed everything; she saved the letters announcing their imminent return. One soldier wrote continually as he got closer to Wisconsin; the last letter was from a hotel in Chicago, where his overtures were answered by her longhand. She was being courted by and would eventually marry a young officer named Harold Allen Zillmann.

Harold came from what Marion deemed a good family. He was a descendant of Ethan Allen, the Revolutionary War hero, and his family had founded a savings and loan company in Thorpe, Wisconsin. He was a determined young man who had pursued Marion despite and throughout her first engagement.

Marion went east and got married in New York. The couple moved to Douglaston, Queens, a spit of land jutting into Long Island Sound. It was a quiet little community laced with maple trees and surrounded by thick marshes. Marion did not bring much more than her boxes of letters, the telegram, and her college degree from the Stout Institute. Harold brought his favorite desk. Both of them were orderly and reserved, and they were comfortable alone. Eventually they made friends with an older couple down the street, and Marion started her garden. She was pleased with the first signs of pregnancy and immediately became easy with her new role. She savored the planning with tender selfishness and designed and sewed brightly colored maternity dresses for herself. Harold was at first confused and mildly defensive about the shift in her attention, but with her precise sense she began sewing him smoking jackets and included him in her project of painting the nursery.

Marion could make an effort, despite her nagging sensation that things weren't quite right. Some of her letters to her first fiancé had been saved and sent back to her, and as she reread them she was always surprised that she had never considered that he might be buried in France and that things might not turn out as she had planned. Except, of course, that Harold was the name of her first fiancé and of the man she had married, and she thought there was something to that. She preferred it when there was "something to" things. She was a practical girl with a good education and could not believe that anything, however small, was without meaning.

The colors of her flowers in her garden in Douglaston were repeated in the amethyst that she wore on her right hand, in the clear red glass dishes in her kitchen, and in the Aztec patterns of yellows in her bathroom. She had no use for pale shades. What she grew in her garden in Douglaston became pressed-flower pictures or flat bouquets, in miniature, under glass in a collection of frames bought at antiques stores. Smaller flowers became the corner decorations under plastic pieces used for place mats. The thickest books in the house were stacked sideways, with wax paper between the pages — here, a collection of Shakespeare secretly drying pansies, an atlas of the world for the greens.

She would snip the lace off her old slips and transform it into flouncy lingerie for the dolls of children she knew. Later, she did it for her daughter, and then for her grandchildren, my sister and me. Everything was orderly. Sentiment was orderly, and people were, above all, polite.

As she continued planting in the crisp November air, her pains became more frequent. She finished the straight row of tulip bulbs — reds, her favorite color, and yellows for the house. She fed the dog and she called her husband. She wanted to make one stop on the way, but Harold said no, so she never got to vote for Herbert Hoover. Instead, that day, she had a baby girl, my mother.

When the baby was born there was some difficulty with the name. Everyone on Harold Zillmann's side of the family had Allen in the name, after Ethan Allen. But Marion Rollins had no use for middle names. She said that they clutter up a signature and give rise to nicknames. The couple decided on the name Allene, and a month after she was born Harold planted a fat pine tree at the end of the yard — a first Christmas tree, the height of the man who planted it and as tall as the peak on the roof of the playhouse he built to keep it company.

The playhouse was just the size for tea for three. Inside, there were sturdy scalloped corner cupboards and curtains to hide the secret meetings of the kids on the block. The back of the peaked house faced a soft brown marshland, and sometimes the tide would flood the playhouse. Out would come the Christopher Robin boots up to the knees, and the pack of young pals would "tut tut" and sweep out the reeds and scoop up the black mud.

There was a hen house where Allene and her friend Elise Linder raised bantam roosters and bunnies. Elise lived up the street, and the girls' fathers were best friends.

Family life was serene, and when Marion made her yearly trip to Wisconsin to visit relatives, the letters from Harold revealed a sincere longing for the company of his wife and daughter and related the smallest details of the weather, his job, and his household activities. It was as though he never wanted her too far away. The details kept them together. He was as particular about details as was his young wife, and he enjoyed and frequently discussed with her the care she took in every aspect of domestic life. He was proud of her, and she thought that his ability to admit it was a fine, but rare, quality in a man.

She was a brilliant cook, stuffing minced dates and nuts into impossibly shaped meringues and creating birthday cakes shaped and colored like the mallards that summered on their wide lawn, which sloped toward the marsh. Marion taught her canary to sing on cue — the same canary she had carried into the Little Church Around the Corner in New York when she and Harold were married. It had sung throughout the service. She was tremendously proud of her abilities and thought it logical to be so. She was more than able; she was talented.

As Allene grew, her parents would sometimes talk about having another child. But they decided that Allene was enough — a beautiful girl with a round face and soft curls who was the precious audience to her father's protective commands and the precious cargo he carried in his arms while whispering his family history. The adventures of the Green Mountain Boys in those woods of New England, liberating Fort Ticonderoga, riding through the towns, and alerting the residents, enthralled the child. Time and time again he would repeat the stories and then carry her up the narrow stairs and have her run her small hands over the smooth wood of the desk that Ethan Allen built, the desk built without nails, stuffed like a mailroom with papers from the phone company, where Harold worked.

Allene's ancestors came to America in 1674 with a trading company from England. They settled first in Connecticut and then branched out as far west as Wisconsin. Several of the boys fought in the Civil War, and there are letters and journals and a family tree, preserved, like her flowers, by Grandma Zillmann.

"It's a good thing to know where you come from," she liked to say, "and just who it is you are marrying."

James Pilkington Roach was twenty-one years old when his future mother-in-law gave birth to his future wife. He was a tall redhead with long straight legs, and he was covered with freckles.

He lived with his parents in Manhattan. They had moved around the city, living at one time in the Rockaways and then over a stable on the East Side. But his favorite home had been an apartment across from the Museum of Natural History. He explored the vast museum every day after school and witnessed the painting of some of the famous habitat murals behind the animals of Asia, Africa, and the United States. He had a passion for Africa, especially for the cats.

James graduated from the High School of Commerce, where he learned shorthand and typing, and four years later he graduated from New York University, where he learned the skills he would use as a newspaperman. Five months after graduation, amid the spring breezes and the expanse of the Green Meadow Golf Club in Westchester, James Roach met Joe Nichols. Joe mistook the lean redhead for one of the players. The youth had the appearance of having been standing around for a while, and he was trim and had an air of buoyant enthusiasm. Clearly, not a reporter. Joe of the *New York Times* introduced himself to Roach of the *New York World*, and the youth began an afternoon of looking at the *Times* reporter somewhat quizzically. The *Times* reporter had been somewhat tardy. Finally the young man said, "I'm surprised you're so late, and you're covering for the *Times*. I've been here since nine this morning."

Thus began a friendship, of the type that enhances lives. Joseph Nichols, who was christened Giuseppe Fappiano, and Junior, as Joe called my father, were both at the *Times* by 1931. The "kid" was a copy reader, and both men worked until after midnight. They shared New York in the daytime and until dawn. Joe introduced my father to the Lower East Side, and many days before work they would walk until they got hungry, eat pasta, walk, and then eat again. Giuseppe Fappiano began to say that James Pilkington Roach was more than part Italian, and the kid agreed.

Together they rode the night boat up the Hudson and went to the racetrack in Saratoga, not infrequently pooling their pocket change on the nose of a filly and winning the fare home. They would share the newspaper on the morning route back to the city, hunched over the sports scores and exchanging winks over the escapades of Legs Diamond in the Catskills as they would plan which speakeasy to drop into that night. Years later they would drape their children over the wide knees of the famous restaurateur Toots Shor, and we'd clutch lamb chops in our fists while Toots told us about our fathers.

My father rarely told stories about himself and would be embarrassed by the tales of him. He believed that quoting yourself was wrong, like loud clothing. He wasn't selfish with his stories; he was quiet with his knowledge. It was always from other people that we would hear about my father putting on skates and practicing with the girls after the *Ice Follies* in the old and towering Madison Square Garden. When he went off to World War II with the Navy, they held his spot on the chorus line. He was a damn good ice skater.

To hear stories from Allene and about her, you had only to ask. For her, the center of attention was the winner's circle; that's where you would wind up if you did things right. All her stories were told as escapades, as larks, starting with her favorite childhood games. She always played a revolutionary, a pirate, an adventurer, although she secretly marveled at her mother's abilities to cook and to sew — to be a mother. The inevitability of children was as attached to the back of Allene's mind as certainly as her unruly hair was shoved into the back of her blouse, but for a while Allene wanted escapades, not dolls.

She was a tomboy as a child, and when she grew and was harnessed into flouncy dresses sewed by her mother, she would pluck off the taffeta flowers from her shoulder straps as soon as she was out the door on the way to her first dances.

At one of her first yacht squadron dances, one of the older men in the community got a bit fresh with her. He was dancing too close and pressing too hard, but she didn't push him away. She kept dancing, somehow transfixed by his crude laugh; then, when she was in a panic at his touch, she heard a young man's voice say, "That, sir, will be about enough of that." She looked up into the face of a new neighbor, who cut in on the intoxicated older man, took Allene's hands, finished the dance with her, and then returned her to her parents' table. She never forgot the romance of being rescued.

With her friends she cut school to go hear Frank Sinatra uptown. With two other girlfriends she ran naked down a back road in Douglaston, and in college she fell in love with a dark and handsome man with whom she read books about the Jazz Age. She fancied herself a sweater girl who pined — and tried — to be a flapper.

My father had dated a Miss America who was terrified of cats, and Joe dated a redhead, Helen, called Nellie. Junior had dated her first, but Joe married her, and the kid was the best man.

When Jim met Allene at the racetrack — he forty-one and she twenty — it was love at first sight. He was running his long fingers through his hair, staring at the blank sheet in his typewriter, and she was having a tour of the press box. She was a cub reporter, and he was the last one left in the hot seat. The other reporters were on the phones, calling in their stories.

He looked up, gasped, was introduced, gasped again, and continued running his fingers through his red hair. The story was tough enough, but with her on his mind it became very delayed. That crisp, sunny day Allene was the perfect foreground figure on Jim's favorite stage, the beauty standing in front of the racetrack. Several years earlier Jim had seen a "done-up" version of his idea of perfection; he had seen Elizabeth Taylor, casually draped against a fence at Belmont racetrack. It was between races, and she was, for the moment, out of the center of attention. He had told Joe that he had never seen a more beautiful sight than Miss Taylor at ease. He told me the same thing years later, but he paused and then smiled and remembered in that perfect private way, and added, "Until I saw your mother."

Allene had a wonderfully casual beauty. Just the way she could toss out phrases and be clever, so she could throw on a dress and look splendid; no make-up, no hype. She was long and curious and had the look of not being easily amused.

He called her three years later. He called Joe next and told him to come to meet his girl at the tennis matches at Forest Hills; Joe and Nellie lived around the corner from the stadium. On that sunny day, as Joe approached, there, at the center of the curve in the top row, was a tall red-haired man with a girl in his arms.

"That was it," said Joe, then a boxing writer, to his friends about Junior, then a turf writer. "I got knocked out in the thirty-ninth round," he said of his marriage at thirty-nine to Nellie, "but Roach got haltered to the altar in the forty-fourth."

He had finally gotten around to asking Allene to marry

him one day in Central Park after she had played him against another sportswriter from the *Long Island Star Journal.* The rivals were the same age — each twenty-one years older than Allene — but the other man had been married and divorced. Allene thought he was a thrill, though he drank too much. Jim she thought respectable, and she went off to Europe to make up her mind. Any commitment, to Allene, was a dare, and this one required dramatic action. She left her itinerary with both men, and at every port there were letters from each asking her to come home. When she did, she had made her decision.

The couple got married in the Little Church Around the Corner, like her parents. There was no canary this time and there were only two witnesses — for her, Elise, with whom she had raised roosters, and for him, of course, Joe Nichols — and her parents and his father.

My mother wore blue.

They left almost immediately for Florida, where Jim would spend the racing season at Hialeah and Allene would learn more about the track. The working honeymoon took place in the Robert Clay Hotel in Miami, and the management did everything to delight the young bride. On her arrival she was presented with a box of pale gray stationery embossed with her name in scarlet letters.

She met the world's greatest sportswriters of the time, and became particularly enchanted with the modest charm and remarkable mind of Red Smith. She learned the difference between the brash sports reporter and the patient and exacting storytellers, like Red, like Jim. She fine-tuned her taste to the delicate snobbery of the best reader, all the while basking in the attention paid to her new husband by the press agents of the track and by the members of the racing association.

On the day she called her "twenty-third anniversary of marriage," she wrote to her parents that "the mink stoles and twenty carat rings flowed like water" in Miami, that she had the sweetest husband anyone ever had (except you, Father)," and that she could not get accustomed to how proud Jim was of her. Her mother decided that she had made a fine choice.

Allene went through her first pregnancy cautiously. She didn't feel right in the role. She walked with care. She took to wearing turbans around her hair, which she pinned up. She wanted to be less glamorous — only for the nine months — but she couldn't quite hide her spectacular legs and her coaxing eyes. Her long slender feet and her agile hands seemed to match the quickness of her laugh, which coincided with the last syllable of a punchline — anticipatory and fast, unlike her image of the proper pregnant woman.

Jim wanted to name the first child Porterhouse, after a favorite racehorse. Allene let him talk about it at parties, but knew that she would prevail. If the baby was a girl, she planned to name her for Jim's deceased mother. Margaret was born on June 10, 1954, two days before the Belmont Stakes. My mother was happy; she got the name she wanted for her daughter. Porterhouse did not win the race; High Gun ran away with it. My father was happy; he tacked on the nickname without an objection. Margaret High Gun Roach was happy, too, when, several years later, she learned that she had had a ten-dollar bet on the big horse.

Beginning with her birth, and throughout her life, my sister went first — the first child, the cue ball to break the rack.

In the beginning my mother was very uncomfortable with motherhood. She would stand over the crib and stare at Margaret when the infant lay crying. Many times Grandma Zillmann had to pick up the baby to prove to Allene that the child would not break. Margaret was a small baby, and Allene was afraid that she might drop her. Grandma Zillman gently tried to teach her daughter that the infant could be made happy with a touch, a simple amusing gesture. Allene remained unsure.

It snowed the day I was born, in the beginning of April 1956. My sister was almost two years old. My first day in the house, my sister was sitting on two phone books at the kitchen table, mimicking in miniature the project my grandmother had before her. When Grandma made cream puffs, Margaret made tiny ones. When Grandma made a dress for Margaret, Margaret used the scraps to make a hat or a shirt for Iggy, her black and white bear whose nose got bitten off one night early in his life. Now, Margaret was using the dull scissors with plastic finger holes. Grandma was using the pinking shears. They were binding the satin edge to the baby blanket Grandma had made for me, Margaret's new sister.

My mother came to the top of the stairs, holding me in her arms. My sister pulled her fingers through the holes in the scissors, slid off the phone books, went to the bottom of the staircase, looked up, and said with the firmness of a two-year-old, "Put her down," then turned on the heel of her Mary Jane and walked away.

I was a big baby, and my mother soon became accustomed to handling me. As I got older, she allowed me to climb and jump off things, when she would warn Margaret against doing the same. The freedom resulted one night in my imitating a circus act I'd seen on television and splitting open the skin next to my right eye. When her mother scolded her for permitting the acrobatics, my mother replied that I was a "durable kid," an expression she used about me for years to come.

Chapter 3

"GIRLS, now let's be Emily-Post-ish," my grandmother loved to say. I hated the words. It was said to both of us, but it was directed to me. I was the one who stopped traffic by sitting in the tar smack in the middle of the newly paved street and to whose duff (my father's word for bottom) the turpentine was applied. I was the one who got caught for daring the next-door neighbor to suck on the end of the tailpipe. And for shaving the dog.

Margaret was Emily-Post-ish. She still is. She could stay clean through a mud fight. I could get filthy in a shower.

My sister listened attentively to my grandmother's gentle speeches on cleanliness. I never thought my grandmother had very much to say to me. But my sister saw past the sagging arms and the large patent leather pocketbooks, the smell of powder and perfume in the tiny bottles from France. Margaret saw a pretty girl with a history. Margaret had managed to tease out the details of the young girl in Wisconsin with the fiancé who had been killed in France, and she had listened to every word. She carefully memorized the lineage of each delicate spoon in the collection on the thick wooden racks in the dining room, to the recipe for meringues and the proper way to sit, while my mother and I would squirm. It became apparent to us early that Grandma Zillmann must have tried the same routine with my mother. It hadn't worked the first time and it certainly wasn't working with me. I took my cues from my mother that all this stuff was for other people. Or, at least, for another type of girl.

My mother and I would slip into the kitchen and eat the peanut butter out of the jar, thrusting crisp apple slices into it. We would wash our hair with Ivory soap if there was no shampoo, standing together in the shower after a family swim at a local pool, and we would giggle and fret and pinch under the table when Grandma gave us lectures. When my grandmother said "Girls," she meant my mother, my sister, and me.

My father, though a turf writer, rarely placed a bet— at least not after he got married. He loved horses. He had a memory for dates, names, weights, and times. He also had a little black book. No girls. Horses. Breeding, interviews, heights, everything on every horse he ever wrote about.

He was tall and distinguished, and going to the races with him was an elegant adventure. Ladies wore hats, and I managed to keep clean. There was an invisible stamp for the back of your hand that showed up only under an ultraviolet light. It smelled like soap and violets and it got you back into the clubhouse where the Vanderbilts had lunch and where, one day, I slid down an escalator banister and was caught by a sailor in uniform.

There was Max Hirsch, who trained High Gun and bought a new Cadillac every year. His right-hand man was a woman named Tad, who had a loud, stacatto laugh. She designed and sewed the silks for the racing stables. My sister and I each had a King Ranch shirt in which we pretended to be Mandarin maidens or jockeys.

Max and Tad employed a wide, black cook who piled up buckwheat flapjacks in the kitchen at six A.M. while the horses worked out. Max could train any animal to do anything. He had a dog who climbed trees. There was a chicken who thought it was a dog and slept, curled up, with the horses. And there was the best trick, when Max would take a quarter out of his deep pocket and throw it over the barn into the woods, and, within moments, back would come a dog with the quarter in its teeth.

In the winter we drove to Hialeah. In the summer, it was Saratoga. My mother's job was to feed my father coffee from a plaid Thermos with a chipped red plastic cup for a top and to keep the "monsters" quiet. We were the black hole in the back seat. Under her seat, my mother would keep a surprise bag — a shiny brown paper bag with toys from the Virginia Variety, the local five-and-ten. It was like feeding time at the zoo. As the ruckus rose, she would toss a puzzle. If there was pinching going on, over would come a kaleidoscope; a bubble-maker for a bite. We nickel-and-dimed her practically to death with bad behavior.

Always, at the end of those long drives, when we would scrape off the ice cream and pick the jacks out of our hair, there would be Grandpa Roach, who had gone ahead alone and would stay for the season. Grandpa Roach was a notorious horseplayer. He bet our ages — my sister's and mine — in the daily double. He drank two half-cups of tea every morning, the top half of each made up of Scotch. He smoked his cigar until it scorched his nails, and then would stuff the stub in a pipe and smoke it till it was ashes. As he got older, he stayed in New York but went to the track almost daily. He took the bus. He was eighty-seven before he accepted a ride from friends.

Grandpa was John Lewis Roach. He was from Liverpool and had come over and fought in the Golden Gloves. He sent for his girl, Margaret, and married her in New York. He looked like a bulldog and he raised blue-tongued chows. He was a chauffeur for Al Smith. One day when he was playing poker with the other drivers, someone ran out of money and threw a gold and diamond ring onto the discards. Grandpa won. He wore the ring for the rest of his life, and when I went off to college he pulled me into his room off the kitchen in our house and told me that when he died he wanted me back there to get that ring off his finger before the undertaker came. He died when I was a fresnman. I never take off that ring.

After a dinner of stewed lamb shanks, he would smooth the wet bones of every shred of meat and place them between his fingers and play them, the percussion, on the table, and he would sing:

> "My girl's a corker, she's a New Yorker.
> I buy her everything to keep her in style.
> She's got a pair of hips just like two battleships.
> Hey, boy, that's where my money goes."

My grandfather's money never went anywhere but under his mattress or out of his pocket and under the grille of a betting window.

At one point he drove for Mr. Cullman of the Philip Morris family. The Cullmans had an estate on Long Island, and Mr. Cullman was rather good at the stock market. One day he leaned forward in the car and said, "John, I don't know how you are set financially, but if you have any money at all, put it in a stock called Pepsi-Cola. It's selling for five cents a share."

My grandfather nodded.

Three weeks later Mr. Cullman again leaned forward in the car for a discussion of high finance. "I hope you've seen the papers, John," he said.

Nod.

"And I hope you bought that stock when I told you."

No nod.

"It's up to seventy-five cents a share now and you ought to buy some more."

"What?" my grandfather barked. "Pay seventy-five cents for something today that I could have had for five cents three weeks ago? Never."

My first memory is of sitting on the beach in Key Biscayne, Florida, during the racing season, probably in the winter of 1959. My mother and I are huddled together. She is pointing to a man who is dark and stooped, and who walks down the beach every morning with another man who is also dark. The one with the stoop is named Nixon, and I remember that my mother gave me my first lesson in government: senators, governors, crooks.

"He's a bad man," my mother said.

I didn't know any bad men yet. I was fascinated.

"He's a bad man. He cheats on his wife."

Grandpa always said that you couldn't cheat at the races as a bettor unless you went to a bookie. So I figured Mr. Nixon went to a bookie. And I decided that his wife must own a track.

I was five when we got a piano. I wanted desperately to play. We took lessons. When the scales and finger exercises became small waltz-tempo melodies, the sister who wasn't playing would stand on the toes of my father's long, wing-tipped shoes, and jaggedly step around the living room, past the Magnavox, over the dog named Saratoga, and sweep into the kitchen, learning to dance.

Piano lessons were bad, but practicing was worse. It was then that my mother became the animal trainer. What Max could do with animals, my mother could do with daughters, luring our wild spirits out of the jungle gym, into the living room for scales. As we moved on to real compositions, our parents would pick out favorite tunes they wanted us to learn.

I grew up thinking that "When I Take My Sugar to Tea" was a popular contemporary song — that and "Deep Purple," whose copyright on my sheet music reads 1934. As a result of my parents' tastes, I played the best whorehouse piano of any kid my age. Joe Nichols was great encouragement. He could play, and sing every word of, "Tea for Two," and he taught me that if you hit a few notes on the top and a few in the bass and sang your lungs out to his favorite, or perhaps "The Sheik of Araby," you were bound to succeed. I lost a lot of sleep through the years, performing at the cocktail parties in our living room, and it wasn't until I was in high school that I realized I didn't know a song written after 1940.

Most of the songs came from my mother's records. She had a collection of leather books with thick paper slips inside for 78s. She had hundreds of records. Each book contained sixteen separate discs and each had a square label glued near the center with her name and the title, written in her script. Along with those she had complete collections of Ella Fitzgerald, Frank Sinatra, and Billie Holiday, just to mention some of the famous names. And she knew the life stories of all the artists as if she had played with them.

Some of the happiest moments of my life were spent kneeling down, flipping through records, and listening to her trace the history of Pee Wee Russell, for instance, through the thirties, through his days with Eddie Condon, playing with Zooty Singleton, through the forties with Bob Haggart, and up to Russell's death, in 1967. I always thought she had a time line of music in her and that every memory was accompanied by a song, a singer, or a bass.

It seems to me that I took piano lessons forever. Margaret dropped them after a couple of years.

I would hear over and over, throughout my life, that my sister had dropped something. I would hear it from my mother, who would tell me that it was my fault, that as soon as I started something, Margaret would become discouraged. She would blame me for what she described as Margaret's "lack of enthusiasm" and, in the same day, ask me whether I'd learned the score of *Carousel.*

When I was about five I developed large blotches all over my body. The pediatrician told my mother that he thought I had leukemia. My mother became frantic. Within a week, the blotches were diagnosed as some form of hives, an extreme allergic reaction to something. The doctor had been very irresponsible in suggesting such an extreme illness, but apparently my mother had insisted on knowing what he was looking for. She told me the story frequently as I was growing up, and she carted me off for blood tests at the slightest provocation. The story always made me feel special — that she was afraid of losing me.

When I was seven, my mother talked the swimming coach into allowing me to compete. I was young, but I loved to swim. Margaret was on the team. We could go together without the danger that we would compete against each other. Or so I thought.

The competition was constant. Height, weight, grades. Swimming, sailing, tennis, piano, friends, freckles.

I was eight when my mother wangled a "ringer's" position for me on a Catholic Youth Organization swimming team because it was one of the best in the city. We were Lutherans. That year we moved to Douglaston, four blocks from the house where my mother had grown up. Four blocks from the first Christmas tree, which now towered over the house and the playhouse. Four blocks from where Grandma Zillmann had recently moved into an apartment building with other widows, who were always off to Hawaii, Copenhagen, church.

We moved into a tall house with a trap door and stained-glass windows of St. George slaying the dragon and St. Joan riding a horse. There were ships and parrots on the windows downstairs. I was crazy about St. Joan. There were hedges taller than my six-foot father and molding around the high ceilings in every room. In the master bedroom there was a chandelier of real crystal that made a great noise when I smacked it with a broom and there were broad wood beams in the ceiling of the dining room.

But best of all, there was a girl next door who was a terror. Priscilla Margaret Anne Elizabeth Dixon could get filthy in a shower, too. At least she could until she turned thirteen and her mother had gotten the rest of the children "raised right" and threw her full attention to cleaning up Priscilla. But for a while we had mud fights and fist fights and knocked out our teeth and smoked cigars under her canopied bed and raised our own brand of suburban hell. In the very beginning, I was just wild about Priscilla.

And my room. Finally, my own room. Priscilla and I had rooms exactly opposite each other and a window-to-window string with a basket attached for messages that went back and forth late into the night. That was the first beauty of having my own room. That and my privacy; no more hiding my sister's Christmas present in our shared closet, where she hung her new clothes and I hung those dreaded hand-me-downs. I hated the system of inheriting clothing, which, I quickly learned, was not to stop in a new house. But at least I had a room of my own.

My mother would wake me up each morning. She would sit on the right side of my antique spool bed and tell me, every morning, as if I could have forgotten it from the day before, to live each day as if it were my last. It was a ritual. Don't look back, she said. When something fails, it's over. When something succeeds, it's done. When something flounders, it's doomed to fail, so get out quickly, just like sleep, when it's over, get up, so get up now.

I always thought that she had just come from giving my sister the same speech. My sister has told me since that she hadn't.

Maybe I was eight when I started water-skiing. I may have

been seven. We were in New Hampshire. Lake Winnipesau-kee. There was a candy store in town as big and deep as a hotel. There were orange salamanders after the kind of rain that can take the edge off even the heat created in a valley.

My swimming had progressed. I had muscles like a clam, hubcaps for knees, and height. And I wanted to learn to water-ski. It looked like fun when my mother did it. She looked as if it made her heart pound. I could tell, when looking back at her on the other end of that slingshot of a yellow line, all legs and breasts and sway and curl of water sliding up from the surface, framing her like a shell, that she wasn't thinking about anything but how good, how clean she felt, and I wanted it too.

I wore my sneakers, over which my mother tightly laced her canvas shoes with the rubber soles. Then came the water-skis. The rubber pockets were vast around my slats of feet. The shoulders of the life jacket kept riding up over my ears; it was the orange-canvas type and it was stiff and cold in the wind, but there I was, on the end of that dock, and there was nothing I wanted to do so much as make that water curl up behind me, next to me, in that Caribbean blur of a blue shell, like her.

My mother sat on the dock on the lake in New Hampshire with her long feet latched into my armpits. I remember seeing just the tips of her red-painted nails peeking out under my arms. She was holding me up in the water to give me "a fighting chance" and she talked to me, running through everything that could happen to me "out there," telling me to remember to lean back and not to bend forward, to watch out for the wake but not to be afraid of it, but if I got near it, not to hesitate, to run right over it, fast. When the boat was out far enough and the line was fully taut, she pulled her stomach muscles and lifted her knees and lifted me from the water for that split second before the pull of the boat took over, and I was gone and then she stood at the end of the dock and yelled, "Stand up! Stand up!"

I remember when she gave up water-skiing. She said she had hurt her back, and I remember how she smiled, years later, when I was fully grown and made her sit on a beach in Barbados and showed her that I had learned to get up on one. She watched me as I came around to finish, dropped the rope, glided right into the sand, and, still moving, ran out of the ski and up to her, and she stared at the water, shaking her head just a little, and said that she had never "quite gotten that right." Dripping wet, I looked down at her and thought that it was the first time I had ever done something she hadn't.

I still love to water-ski. I love to start on one and pull and fight my way out of the barrel of water that curls in front of me from the pressure. Water-skiing and sailing small boats, close to the water, at great speed in a dark day's wind make me laugh out loud.

We sailed a great deal together. She got me a boat when I was thirteen, and I raced and sailed and mooned around the same dock she had as a girl. One night a week in the summers, we would race together. Hunched down, eating tuna fish sandwiches, delicately adjusting the sheets and the sails, we would race my Blue Jay and she would tell me about her Nimblet, which she raced at my age. Her boat was lost in a hurricane when a friend didn't tie it up correctly, "so always tie it this way," she would tell me, demonstrating, "the way I did when I was your age." At my age. But she was my age. She was with me and she was racing with me and we were in blue jackets and we were wet and when the wind would pick up and the boat would heel way over, we balanced on the rail, with our toes tucked into the centerboard trunk, and we leaned way out, over the water, over the evening, daring the water to curl up and get us. She would be in front, the first to get wet. I would steady the tiller, inching us closer to the wind, a delicate balance of love and speed. And we laughed and whooped when the wind backed around and tossed us into the cabin. We got a lot of bruises on our matching kneecaps. We were pals.

Somewhere between the ages of nine and ten Margaret started going to our family doctor in New York once a week. My mother took her. Dr. John Prutting had been a close friend of my father's for many years. He became a close friend of the family; he spent time in Douglaston with us, and we spent time on Long Island and in his vast apartment in New York with him. Every week as they'd sit and talk with the doctor — Margaret rarely spoke at the sessions, as noted in the doctor's records — my mother would talk about Margaret's depression. Some weeks it was less severe; some weeks, said my mother, there was real cause for concern. There was a hint of danger in my mother's voice.

Margaret remembers quite clearly going along with this and knowing, even at that young age, that she was not the patient. Margaret knew that Mother was talking about herself. Margaret also remembers that Dr. Prutting always spoke right to my mother about depression, and that Margaret was totally ignored. Dr. Prutting would warn Mother about the dangers of depressed behavior, of the inability to cope with social situations, and she would nod her head solemnly. Eventually, Margaret was diagnosed as a depressive, and an antidepressant was prescribed. She never took the drug. She remembers asking Mother about it and being told not to worry.

That, Margaret recalls, was the only discussion the two of them had about the visits. They never talked about them in the car on the way there or back. Margaret just went along and did her homework in the car and seemed not to care, but, in truth, it was during this period that Margaret began to believe that our mother was very unhappy.

At this very early age Margaret quietly accepted a burden that she only recently has discussed with me. She knew there was something wrong, but, being the eldest child, she thought that it came with the territory, that she had to accept it and do as she was told. She was to act with quiet responsibility — unlike, perhaps, her little sister, who objected to everything, from hand-me-downs to being quiet.

And so Margaret and my mother went into the doctor together, my father paid the bills, but no one ever asked Allene what it was that was troubling her. I never noticed this quiet pact between the two of them and I did not notice that my mother was depressed. I did, however, began to notice at this time the differences between my sister and me.

Margaret was a pale and quiet child. She was a reader. She listened. She didn't like to dance. She liked to give advice. She didn't like sports, and she preferred not to be pushed into lessons. She liked to cook and she loved flowers and antiques and painting. She adored Grandma Zillmann, and together they made pressed-flower pictures and designed birthday cakes for local children; their favorite cake was an elaborately happy face with shredded coconut for hair and M & Ms for freckles. Margaret loved it when Grandma Zillmann baby-sat.

I loved it when Grandpa Roach came and taught us to play poker.

Beginning in our youth, the greatest difference between Margaret and me was our attitude toward our mother. Margaret found her embarrassingly aggressive. I thought she was just the push I needed.

As I approached eighth grade, New York City was battling a long school strike. My grandmother was paying for Margaret to go to a private school. Girls' school. I was to go there in ninth grade. I had seen my sister's uniform. I was in no rush.

For three weeks, while parochial and private school children learned, the rest of us played football.

Another girl going to private school was Priscilla, my neighbor and old pal. We hadn't been friends for a year or so. This was the period when her mother was working her over. Priscilla wore kilts and sweaters, and I thought she was not my type anymore. One night my mother announced that I was to play tennis the very next day with Priscilla. I winced. I didn't want to be caught dead with her in a dark basement, let alone on a tennis court for all my friends to see. My mother insisted.

Standing by the court, I caught sight of this vision in white entering the club. She had pigtails wrapped in thick yarn, a skirt with a blue hem, and as she got closer, I could tell, God forbid, she was wearing a bra. After we played, I said I was going down the street to the dock to go swimming. She said she couldn't go, and I couldn't figure out how a young girl "couldn't" go swimming when she was all hot and sweaty and must, if she was at all normal, be dying to go.

So much for that. Later that night I reported to my mother that she could keep her matchmaking to herself. My sister said that Priscilla seemed like a "very nice girl." It had recently occurred to me that everyone Margaret thought was a nice girl, was, well, quieter than I. That did it.

Several weeks into the school strike, my mother told me that she was going to take me over to the Cathedral School of St. Mary, in Garden City, Long Island, where my sister was, for a test. I did not want to go to a girls' school. Girls were what my sister was. I love my sister dearly, but at the age of thirteen I did not like her much. We had always been different — she baked and gardened while I just grew bruises — but ever since she got breasts, she just wasn't the same old girl at all.

I liked boys. I understood them. I was as tall as they, could run as fast, understood football, played soccer, swam, and sailed with them. And as one by one my girlfriends got breasts — those mysterious life-changing swells of pomposity or shyness — I lost them as friends. Soon, I also started to lose a lot of my male friends to breasts. It was very depressing. I looked like a door and I wanted to look like a door. I discussed it with my mother. My mother had marvelous breasts.

"Growing up is a wonderful thing," she said. "It's a magical mysterious thing, also. Look at your sister; she's growing up."

Ugh. My sister was now at the stage where she locked the bathroom door.

"Boys like girls with breasts." Ever the diplomat.

I was in tears. We were sitting in the den upstairs, all books and dust, and my mother had stopped her work on one of her evening courses. I knew that I did not always get the opportunity of having her undivided attention. Clearly, this was an important subject. When my mother turned her attention to me, I was always enrapt. She had an immaculately intelligent face and she had soft hair. When I was quite young I wrote in a diary, "Never trust a woman whose hair doesn't move," an adage I composed after staring at my mother. I never got used simply to looking at my mother. I was always staring at her beauty, taking an inside look at perfect, unattainable glamour. I always thought she never did anything to it; no hairdos, only a touch of make-up for her. Her face was tight and strong. Her hair was below her shoulders and curled.

So as I sat there that evening, wondering about breasts, looking into her face, I realized that, as had happened so many times before, I was going to get the truth. I didn't squirm. "Don't they get in the way?" I asked.

My mother was a powerful tennis player. No tennis lady, she. She was able to play with the men. She was a force to be reckoned with. "Not really."

I was dismayed. I felt betrayed. I also felt, though, for the first time, that if she had them, then I'd better get them too. It wasn't, I was to discover, as easy as that.

First of all, I was a year ahead in school. I had skipped third grade, which means that to this day I cannot do any arithmetic but addition and subtraction. Not only was I younger than the girls in my grade; I was what was known as "a late bloomer." I was not, as I had overheard one of my friends described, "a garden of heavenly delights."

I started at St. Mary's midway through October. What I had never anticipated was the boundless joy of being with 124 girls at various stages of development. Not everyone had breasts. Many of them played basketball. Many of them had older sisters — with breasts — in the school.

I was the only girl in the eighth grade to make junior varsity basketball. That meant that I stayed after school, and my mother had to drive forty-five minutes every night I stayed. But she was my biggest fan.

I was crazy about my knees. My knees nearly drove my mother crazy. Joe Namath had bad knees, so I decided that I had to have them too. He was my idol. I had an entire wall of my room lathered with pictures of him. And my father had gotten his signature for me. It was my favorite possession. First it was the right knee. It hurt. We tried ice, heat, elastic bandages. Then it was the left one. It got the same treatment. Back and forth we went with remedies and a relentless volley of real and imagined pains.

Growing pains, said one doctor. "Nonsense," said my mother. "This kid loves to grow." My mother explained to me and to him that in some children, growing was not a horror; it was a joy. She was off, on her panegyric to the delight of her own youth, her sailing and tennis. I was there to be the articulation of her youth, the example of the things she was clever enough to say.

Six doctors later, it was cysts in the cartilage. The doctor said he would like to operate.

My mother had the most beautiful legs in America, if not the world. I have heard, and I had heard even at that time, stories about her legs, about the reaction of men to her legs.

"Growing pains," she said to me, changing her mind. "You have growing pains. Live with them. No operations, no scars, not with those legs."

So, growing pains it was. I played basketball with as much fervor as, I imagine, I have ever mustered. She came to every game she could.

I wore a combination of arrangements on my knee, a dead giveaway to the opposition. Once, a girl ran up to me in a game and kicked me squarely on the right kneecap. I was in agony.

My mother flew off the bleachers. I remember the remarkable echo and the screaming and the fact that she never seemed to touch a step. She pulled at the referee and shouted at her. She shouted at the girl. She shouted at me to defend myself.

Later, when the girl was making a lay-up at the opposite end, I applied a little pressure with my sneaker to her ankle. While they carried the wailing and shrieking fifteen-year-old off the court, my mother looked out under her arched eyebrows and gave me the hint of a smile. Her kid. She was competitive as hell.

I talked my way onto the tennis team when I was in ninth grade. Another redhead, named Barbara, had given me the tip that the team needed one more doubles player for a match the next day. I ran over to the gym and pleaded my way on. I swore I was good, and it worked. Late in the afternoon of the match I began to feel dreadful. I had pains in my back and pains in my head. I went to the bathroom. As I sat there, alone in a darkened stall, I remembered my mother's premature lecture, two years before this terrible moment, when she had gotten out the pamphlets, the diagrams, and the encyclopedia.

"If you don't know what it is, where it is, or how to spell it, look it up" was my father's dictum. Never a quick answer. Get out the encyclopedia, the atlas, the dictionary.

Two years too soon, armed with all that embarrassing and, at the time, unnecessary literature, she had explained menstruation. I knew as she explained it that I was nowhere near needing to know the stuff. But now, two years later, I sat in horror in the bathroom, thinking it was a mistake, but of course not remembering a word of it. So I ignored it.

Later it was harder to ignore. I was embarrassed. Too embarrassed, certainly, to ask anyone. Too embarrassed to lean into any of my tennis shots, I lost the match for us.

My mother picked me up after the match. "How was it?"

"Awful. I played miserably."

She was angry. "Why?"

"Why. Um. Well, Oh, God. Ugh, I hate this. God, I hate this. Why didn't you tell me about this?"

She was thrilled. I couldn't believe it. Thrilled.

"You are growing up." She actually hugged me. My mother never hugged anyone. She told me she hated physical contact, especially between women. She said only "silly women" kissed hello. She hated silly women.

My sister, it seemed to me, had just breezed through all this feminine stuff. Overnight she had adopted an appealing insecurity I thought all real "girls" needed to get along with the rest of the world. Margaret noticed things and would cry. She noticed things I never saw. She noticed that our parents had what my mother would tell me only years later was "a lousy marriage."

Margaret witnessed things I sat through and ignored. If there was tension in the house, she was the first to retreat to her room and lock the door. If there was a disagreement at dinner, she would take her plate to the other room while I ate through the disagreement — no matter how large — and seemingly noticed nothing. Margaret was upstairs, considering the rights and wrongs of the conflict, while I thought she was hiding.

My father believed you could build anything with patient care. He believed you could learn after school what wasn't handed to you. The books are always going to be there, he said; just keep reading. It made for a difficult marriage, but one I think I understand. My mother was so very exciting and so very beautiful. She was smart and she was quick and agile, interesting to the point of being compelling. She was also twenty-one years younger than he. He was admirable and consistent, a teacher and a listener. They needed each other desperately but devoured each other's very strengths. My mother disrupted my father's enviable calm, and my father tried to curtail my mother's remarkable enthusiasm. It was not a good case of opposites attracting each other; what had once been an attraction became an annoyance.

Margaret knew this early in her life, and she chose to favor our father. She always thought that our mother was unhappy, and she still believes that the unhappiness came from her never having taken a chance in her life — from marrying a lovely, gentle, secure man, instead of being this intrepid woman she believed Margaret would never be but that I might become. My mother's way with me was, according to Margaret, obsessive. Also, my sister believes that I never saw any of it. She is right. I saw no reason to object to being the focus of my mother's affections and attention; it was just fine with me.

I adored both of my parents. Both of them played basketball with me in the backyard or soccer in the front, and that was what I liked to do. My sister, I thought at the time, enjoyed being a brooder, enjoyed keeping quiet. What she must have been feeling was an excruciating rejection by my mother, which I never sensed. I assumed that they simply didn't get along.

While we were still in our teens, I woke one morning and found that my mother's close friend Lisa was asleep in my father's bed. My father was away on a trip. Margaret was dozing in a chair in our parents' bedroom. I walked in to wake up the bunch, including my mother, and discovered that my mother had fallen down the stairs during the night. That was about all I got out of anyone at the time, and I was angry at the presence of other people in the room; I wanted to talk to my mother. But she was very groggy.

Late the night before, Margaret had found my mother at the bottom of the stairs, semiconscious, quite intoxicated, and with her right calf ripped its full length. She lay bleeding in the hallway. The first thing Margaret had done was slip upstairs and make sure my door was closed. Then she called the doctor and Lisa. It made sense to call her; Lisa and my mother had been friends for many years. They raised their daughters together, played tennis several times a week, and were Girl Scout leaders in the same troop. When there was a problem, it wasn't nearly as odd to see Lisa in our house as it was to see Margaret, slumped and sleeping in a chair. Lisa was forever rescuing one of us when we were locked out or stuck for a ride or needed just about anything. Apparently, the first thing Lisa asked on her arrival was whether I had seen my mother's fall. Margaret said no, and they decided not to tell me. My mother was in on the bargain by the next morning. They weren't going to tell me that my mother got drunk and fell down. I learned the truth years later.

Margaret and I still weren't very close when she went off to college in Kalamazoo, Michigan. Her best friend, Lisa's daughter, Lynn, had gone off to college in Rochester the year before, and ever since, Margaret had really looked forward to going away, too. I imagine that all of those years of believing that she was bearing the brunt of the family problems made her eager to get out. Then, without her very close friend, it all must have been unbearable.

I was glad to get her out of the house. During high school she was critical of me if I smoked cigarettes or sneaked out at night with my pack of friends. She never told on me, but she always let me know that she knew and that she completely disapproved.

She stayed at Kalamazoo for a semester. She was very unhappy with all the snow and moved back home and almost instantly into an apartment in Manhattan. She was just seventeen. Over the next few years she lived in several apartments in the city. Once she lived above a tombstone manufacturer and around the corner from the New York chapter of the Hell's Angels.

At some point in this period my mother wrote to her relatives and described her mother's death. My mother had found Grandma Zillmann dead in her apartment. It was shocking, but some of Grandma Zillmann's friends, gathered later at the funeral parlor, said to my mother that they hoped they would go like that; she had just died one night while getting ready for bed. I don't know why we have my mother's letter, but I found it recently and was struck by her words. She wrote about Margaret only that she was "living in the city and seems happy." She went on to say that I was the captain of my basketball team, the president of the student council, and was happy about going away to college; she described me as a "real doer." It is too simple to say that my mother and sister did not find each other interesting.

Margaret was dating a black man when I was a senior in high school. My mother and father had raised us right. There is no difference between people. My mother's reaction was classic. She didn't dare say a word, with her liberal history, and my father, knowing that she was really uncomfortable with Margaret's choice, frequently smirked at her refusal to admit it. One night Margaret and Doug, her date, took me to a private club where people smoked pot. I remember thinking that night that Margaret was much more interesting than I had ever realized. But I couldn't imagine where she'd learned anything interesting, if not from me.

On her own, Margaret established herself in New York with friends and a job. She visited our father at his job at the *New York Times* but rarely came out to Douglaston, and therefore almost never saw our mother or me. She started weekly therapy at a counseling clinic, something she tried only once to explain to me after I had asked her what the problem was, and she said, "Mommy, but you'll never understand."

I let it drop.

My mother had started working when Margaret and I were in junior high school. She began with volunteer work for the Visiting Nurse Service; then she returned to school. She told me that she owed a great deal of her desire to learn to a woman named Janet Kaplan.

Janet Kaplan was a divorcée from Great Neck, and my mother added with a smile, "She knows about jazz." Together they spent many evenings in Manhattan at Eddie Condon's.

They had met at Nassau County's adult education classes. ("Stupid name," my mother would say; "degrading, as if there's something strange about educating adults, as if those of us who had children weren't children ourselves when we had them and then adults when we had time to get back to school. Stupid name.") Together they ran the gamut of classes: Spanish for beginners, Greek mythology, creative writing, Italian bread, Chinese wokery, and self-awareness.

Once a week for years my mother went off to get to know herself better, and every day she became more fiercely independent. Always there was an evening or two out, as well as the classes. Always it was jazz.

Then Janet moved to Manhattan, and my mother would spend some nights there. Once there was a trip to Washington and then another to New Orleans to hear Dixieland jazz at Preservation Hall.

Before Janet, I think of my mother in loose shirts with that turban, aggressive but domesticated, leaning over the ironing board I used as my hiding place when I played Swamp Fox, the Southern Revolutionary she had taught me about, acting out my fantasy in front of her only. Once Janet Kaplan came into the picture, my mother seemed to have someone else to tell about revolutionaries, and there was someone to spur her thoughts. Suddenly there were museum memberships and openings. Overnight we dusted off and put out the art books and used the fine china.

But Janet Kaplan never came to dinner, and later, when she had her accident, I remember thinking that such an active person as Janet must have been furious to be laid up. She had broken her ankle, and my mother went to stay with her for two weeks. My father told me about the accident. He was aware that she was a compelling force in my mother's life and he seemed glad to have my mother so happy, even if it was outside our home.

I was unaware that he had never met her. I was unaware that Janet did not exist. Margaret knew.

I was a junior in high school when my father first got sick. He had never been ill. In thirty-five years at the *Times*, he never missed a day. He never even got colds. He didn't drink anything but beer. He didn't smoke. First he developed bleeding ulcers and had to have a transfusion. Several months later, at Thanksgiving, he was out raking leaves and came in with a relentless pain in his back. He was hospi-

talized and ready to come home when Dr. Prutting ran a
couple of tests to see why a healthy man in his mid-sixties
cracked a vertebra. He was diagnosed as having multiple
myeloma — cancer of the bone marrow. It had started in
his spine.

A friend of mine told me that my sister had said my father
was quite ill. My mother and sister had known the diagnosis
for two weeks before I confronted them and my mother
admitted that yes, he had cancer. I was very angry with both
of them. And very confused. I never knew that I was unaware of anything in the house, and I did not suspect that
there was more.

By the time we were in high school, my mother's initial
desire to fill time had become a fierce determination to work.
She decided to get a master's degree in education from New
York University. My mother said that Janet Kaplan was getting one, too.

The tennis ladies took it badly. She wasn't available for
Ladies' Day anymore. She started teaching part time at a
Montessori preschool on the Lower East Side of New York
and attending classes. My mother completed her master's
while I was in college and immediately began teaching full
time at the school downtown. She made ninety dollars every
two weeks. She got up at 5:45 A.M. and drove to the city.
My father wrote me about those mornings. It was then that
he started the letters that I call the "cat series."

Notes from the cats appeared, all in lower case because
it was impossible for paws to reach from the shift key to the
letters without losing balance. Kittens on the keys. I would
read the letters aloud to my roommates.

november 15, 1976

dear marion —

you do not know me but i feel that i know you. i have
heard your parents talk about you and that is why i feel

that i know you. maybe i should introduce myself. i am called 5½ cat by your father. i live in your house. let me explain — i have taken up light housekeeping in the garage and last week your mother started getting sorry for me and putting out food for me and at that point your father said oh me now we have 5½ cats, and so he named me 5½ cat. actually my name is ethelbert.

The letter goes on, with a sketch done by a cat named coley who is really named Coleman Hawkins, for the saxophonist, and in whose name I had taken a subscription to *The New Yorker* and had it sent to the house in Douglaston. That was when the letters started; coley wrote to thank me.

I loved my father's eccentricity. I loved his calm. I loved my mother's strength. She was working on the corner of Houston Street and Avenue D, which is not a safe neighborhood. But she loved the children. Though some of the stories she brought home were wonderful, my mother in the slums was not just a self-righteous suburban woman assuaging her guilt. She cared.

She had a strained and jump-started commitment to the education of the children. She would go on home visits, up collapsing staircases, where mothers were sixteen and there were no fathers to be found. She would walk into fights that fitted no notions I had of "domestic violence," and she would see needles and nickel bags, and she would drive home in a rage. But she always got up the next morning before six and she always went in and I admired her tremendously.

I visited the school many times. Spending the day there was exhausting and, for me, depressing. But she was determined. The class brat — the one who tore up the paintings of others, threw his food, and at four and a half swore like a boxer — leaned up to her one day and spat in her face. Without missing a beat, she spat right back. Instant respect. From then on, he napped in her arms.

That was the way I knew her then.

Chapter 4

I GREW UP thinking that parents often took separate vacations. Our parents had religiously taken us on family vacations when we were younger — the islands, a dude ranch in Colorado, Mexico — but as we got into our teens, we had individual tastes, which everyone respected, and we went in pairs — my father and I went to Barbados for ten days — or alone, as my mother had gone camping on St. John. It wasn't new, really. It had started when my father had covered the Olympics in Tokyo in 1964 and then had gone around the world from there.

Traveling was a big thing in our family. By the time I was in college — at St. Lawrence University, in upstate New York — I had the pattern down: go if you possibly can and go almost anywhere. I had traveled to Canada a great deal when I was in college, but by my junior year I was truly antsy.

I spent Thanksgiving of my junior year as always, eating. We were at the dining room when I announced — most specifically to my father — that I had applied for and had been accepted to go to East Africa for a semester. Next semester. My father looked startled.

It was my mother's plan, that I should get accepted for

the trip before mentioning it to Daddy. She had told me to "get the message across as early as possible," but I had procrastinated. The trip was to start in January. My mother, however, was ready for a fight. I was going; that was it. She, she told me, would be in Egypt while I was there. She had yet to tell my father. It occurred to me that I was breaking the ice.

I had never wanted to go to Europe. I knew that I would get there; I knew that it would be pretty. I had always wanted to go to Africa. My father had given me books on it when I was about ten. I read and reread them. And then I made my plans. Finally, at nineteen, I had found a way, and since I hadn't mentioned it yet, my mother dropped an unmistakable hint at dinner. I had to ask.

The program would take me to Nairobi for four months, I explained. He looked at me over his half-glasses and over his drinking glass. He put down his drinking glass. He relaxed his face. "No baby of mine is going to Africa," he said. That, he thought, was that. Two months later, equipped with everything Abercrombie and Fitch could sell my wonderful father, I was off.

My mother had taught me to be a precise athlete, a competitive person, and something of an optimist. But the thing she did best was to set me up for my first love.

There was one rule: he had to be Erroll Flynn. Not the Erroll Flynn of real life, but the Erroll Flynn of the movies — before he got fat. He had to be daring, bright, cunning, romantic, tall, forceful, adventurous, brave, and something of a masher. James Bond would do.

I thought I had found the right young man, once. Before that, even I realized the limitations of the eclectic pack I had dated: too short, too meek, attractive but boring. Most of the time I went to great lengths to keep them from meeting my mother. She was brutal about boyfriends. She believed that they were an important commodity. This one was the first young man I had been dying to have meet her. I thought he had everything. I invited him to the house, and she met him, sat with him for five minutes, and then asked him to excuse us.

Into the kitchen we went. "Well," she said with a grand sweep of her voice, "you have outdone yourself this time. He looks like Erroll Flynn minus the sword and," in a voice that echoed grinding glass, "he's the most vapid young man I've ever met."

Oh, well.

Two months later, I was sitting alone on the bench at the airport, contemplating my fate. I was nineteen years old and something less than worldly. I was to spend ten days in London before joining the group for four months in Kenya. I was proud of myself, but nervous, almost over-weight in that junior-in-college-in-hiking-boots way, and hopelessly romantic.

I was engrossed in my hands, but when I looked up from my cuticles I saw a tall, graceful man in a full-length fur coat parading an extraordinarily pretty woman to the gate. He was lightly touching her under the forearm, and they were chatting softly, and I could see that his hands were broad and strong and that from under a crisp suit jacket, under that coat, peeped a white shirt cuff, stiff as good paper. He made it look as if she were important cargo. He was delivering her, and I thought that she, at that moment, was the luckiest woman in the world.

There was the confusion of the embarkation. I followed his coat with my eyes. I followed the broad, thick chest and the careful attention he was paying to the woman. I felt awkward. I went to the ladies' room and washed my face, smoothed my clothes, and put on make-up. I didn't want to be nineteen anymore. I wanted to go on an adventure.

I boarded the plane, but he was nowhere to be found.

Slumped into my seat, tennis racquet in hand, I was shaken from my dismay by a young man in revoltingly tight trousers and a repellent manner. He was loud and flirtatious. He told me that he couldn't wait to get right back and talk to me, but that he was going for a beer, and did I want one. I told him to go to hell, put up the armrest to the seat, and lay down with a sigh, knowing I'd never find Erroll Flynn, never be walked through an airport like that, and never be anything other than nineteen and awkward.

The back of my seat was pulled and I thought, Oh God, this jerk is back already, and I squeezed my eyes shut as, just above me, a voice in a Scottish lilt said, "You make it look as if it's been a long trip already," and I looked up into the most perfect face I've ever known, framed by that fur.

The plane was delayed and then canceled and we were taken by bus into Montreal. I saw him in the lobby the next morning, writing with a flourish on a stack of postcards, laughing out loud to himself, using a gold pen. I slinked behind him, embarrassed to be wearing the same clothes, and then crept away, after catching the warm smell of his cologne and seeing that the ink from his pen was aquamarine.

Later, the passengers were taken by buses to the terminal. I maneuvered myself near him on the bus and then near him on line at the airport. He looked over once and smiled, and I felt what we call the "redhead's revenge" start at my elbows and burn up to my forehead — a drastic blush — and he chuckled. I wanted to perish.

He led the woman, again by the forearm, onto the plane, and they were gone. After takeoff I heard that accent coming up the aisle, singing, "Little darling, it's been a long, cold lonely winter." He stopped and I looked up and he kept singing as he led me back to where they were sitting. The three of us sat up all night, happily drinking from a bottle of Canadian Club, and mostly I listened to his stories about Canada, Scotland, South Africa, and rock stars. She was the wife of his business partner, and they were going first to London and then South Africa, where she and her husband lived. I remember telling them about college — he had never been — and thinking that he was forty.

I thought, when I looked at him, Playboy, he's a playboy, an international playboy, maybe. But he was more complex than that. He introduced himself as Douglas, King of Scotland, and I almost believed him.

He told me he'd drop me at my hotel, but when he got there he didn't like it and told me to shower and be ready in an hour. He came back and took me to lunch in a smoky pub that served slabs of meat and small round glasses of warm beer. He said that he would show me London but that I must pay strict attention. There were rides in the backs of square black cabs and there were quizzes about the Queen Mother and there were long, bantering dinners, and back I would go to my hotel room and be deposited, with a kiss on my forehead. I was "the child," and he was there to look after my safety.

He responded to bits of knowledge — writers, American history — like a cat to a string; he could not leave it alone. His education had come on the streets and he was proud of it, but he adored knowing anything, and it made me feel smart. He was clever, and that made me want to be clever, too.

He lived in a house behind the Regent's Park Zoo that was like a wide brownstone, where I learned to sip a cocktail and was asked about Muhammad Ali and Watergate.

He had an emerald tie tack and creased trousers. No cuffs. I had T-shirts and cotton jeans and only a few very unflattering winter clothes. I was, after all, on my way to Africa. Before I left, my mother had tried to get me to buy some pretty shoes for London and had given me $150, which I had spent on rock-climbing boots. She abandoned the project.

We went to lunch at the inn in the park, he in a Dunhill suit and the fur coat, I in draw-string cotton red trousers, sneakers, and a striped T-shirt.

"Tell the gentleman what you want," he commanded.

"A lobster and the . . ."

"No, tell the gentleman what you really want."

"Hm."

"She wants to be the first female attorney general of the United States."

It was my secret. I thought he was poking fun and I was terribly hurt.

"If you really want it," he said, noticing the scowl, "you have to get used to the idea, believe in it, talk about it, and work for it. Now, what do you want for lunch?"

After lunch each day there was the ride through London and the quizzes: Who lives here? What is the name of this park? Where did? What did? When? I wanted to be under that spell forever.

"Stop here," he said to the cabbie. "You wait," he said to me.

He was thinking of bringing fast-food hamburgers to South Africa, where he was moving. He came back to the cab with a bag of chicken and chips and gave them to the driver.

"Now," he said, leaning up into the cabbie's shoulder, "it's lunchtime."

"Right."

"And you are hungry."

"Yes, sir."

"And you get a bag of chicken and chips."

"Because you bought them, sir."

"But you think, well, my wife will probably have chips for dinner and maybe chicken," said Douglas. He turned back to me. "I'm going to show you, you'll see. They will love this there. They will be killing themselves for it."

I had been arguing for what I thought was the preservation of a beautiful thing, life without fast-food hamburgers.

"They'll love this in South Africa." Back to the cabbie. "So you are thinking you'd rather have something else."

"I am?"

"You'd rather have a hamburger."

The cabbie stopped in traffic. He looked over his shoulder. "You want these back, sir?"

"No, it's just that your wife is going to serve this later, so if you could get a hamburger . . ."

"If I could get a wife, sir."

There were radios built into the bedside table of every hotel I stayed in while in London — I stayed in four hotels in ten days. Douglas kept insisting that I move, that I see the city, live in different sections. And each hotel room had the same bedside table arrangement. I would listen to the one meshed speaker late into the night, after the dinners, after the cab rides, and I would imagine we were dancing.

He'd be dancing somewhere with someone in a gown. I figured he was champagne and orchids at midnight, lightning and leather, and as hot as saxophones at noon. There I was, stretched out in one of my father's pink Brooks Brothers shirts, wishing I had fingernails.

He remembered seeing his father only once in his life, at a funeral: the man who came across the room with a curious look and gave him a five-pound note. He thought at the time that the man was a pretty nice chap. When he was a little older he drew a cartoon lampooning the headmaster, named Wilson, at his school. The character in the strip was named Mr. W, and it was unkind but on the money. The real Mr. Wilson suspected the brash young Douglas but never got a confession from him. Every day another installment would appear on the bulletin board on the main hall, and every day the assembled boys would be grilled. Mr. Wilson never found his culprit, and the kid learned that he could get away with anything.

As he got older and his brother and sister had children, and Eddie, his best friend, and Jenny (the woman on the plane, Eddie's wife) had children, he told them the story of the Black Spinney, which he told to me one night at my doorway. The creature can send children to bed faster than a dose of uneaten Brussels sprouts. The Black Spinney is the most terrifying creature any child — of any age — ever begged to meet at bedtime.

Douglas could wind a story into a web from nothing. Point to a lamppost and learn about its love life with the postbox on the corner; promise to be good just so that fairies dance under the fold the sheet makes when tucked around the blanket. But the best was the Black Spinney — scariest, largest, darkest of all, alive in the cabbage patch, under the stairs, in your sister's closet when she's bad. He told the most beautiful stories to children and he told a lot of them to me.

While he sought his fortune, he bought his mother a house in Scotland and named it Sans Souci. But once a year he transported her to him, and for six weeks she'd be the girl in his life. He told me that he didn't want to be "an entry in a young girl's journal on her first trip to Europe." He told me never to trust anyone who tried to give me his business card. He taught me to say "straightaway" instead of "immediately," and never to say "can't" but to say "won't," and one night he held me an inch off the floor by the throat, a thumb tucked under my chin, and he asked me if I was afraid and I said no and he said I should be and then he slid me down the wall and taught me the proper way to be in love.

. . .

I spent four and a half months in Kenya. I worked on a newspaper that preferred a multiple-victim car accident on the front page to world news. I and others lived in a village on a tea plantation for the first three days — to break us of being tourists — and I saw the morning sun crest the world from the top of Kilimanjaro.

When I came down from a five-day trip climbing Kilimanjaro, there was a letter from my mother that said she had spent the past three weeks cleaning Margaret's room and was about to start on mine.

There are things in every young woman's room that no mother, even Allene the open-minded, should see. I sent off a cable: CLIMBED SUCCESSFULLY. DO NOT CLEAN ROOM PLEASE.

What my mother knew about traveling was not mirrored in her knowledge of geography. While in Nairobi, I called home. I got my father.

"Hello, Daddy?" I said into the phone, stunned at the clear connection.

"Who is that?" he asked, angrily.

"Marion, it's Marion, Daddy, your baby daughter." (I was baby daughter or tingletot.)

"Don't tease me," he snapped. "My baby daughter is in Africa. So is her mother."

I convinced him. We both cried. I missed him so very much. I wanted him to be there with me on my grand adventure. He would have been crazy about the lions.

That day I got a cable from my mother. IN EGYPT IN CAIRO, it read. CAN YOU COME UP FOR THE WEEKEND? I cabled her back. MOM LOOK AT A MAP.

In London, on my way home, I missed my flight to Montreal. I tried to transfer my ticket and was told that because of the excursion fare it was worth only thirty-three pounds. Not good.

I tried to cash a check, but no one would take it. It was midnight, and I was tired and hot and broke and knew three people in London.

My first two calls received no answer. The third was to whoever was living at the house tucked behind the Regent's Park Zoo, for it was to be sold while he was in South Africa, making his fortune.

"What?" was the first thing I heard. "This had better be good."

I recognized the voice, certainly. "Hello," I said.

"Ah," as if it were a trajectory. "Where are you, child?"

"The airport."

"Get here."

"I haven't any money."

"Get here."

Click. Saved again.

I had a bath while in the other room he sang several choruses of "Here Comes the Sun," interspersed with directions on how to bathe, as if I might miss a spot. "Little darling, get those damn elbows, it's been a long, cold lonely winter, behind the knees."

The next day he went to Johannesburg and I went home. I didn't know it, but earlier that night, while walking through London, he had given his last five pounds to a woman begging money.

He didn't tell me, but he was broke. I didn't tell him, but I was in love. Lock, stock, and looks.

My mother was delighted. She said he sounded perfect. She said that if I played it right, someday he'd come and get me. We didn't tell my father.

By the following year, when I graduated from college, Margaret had been at the *New York Times* for three years, first as a copy person, then as a news clerk, and then as a copy editor in the sports department — the only woman copy editor there. By the time I was a junior in college she was writing the women's sports column and one day she helped make a very strong man named Arnold Schwarzenegger very famous in a story on body-building. Perhaps to the rest of the world this sport was legitimate, but to the readers of the *New York Times* it was something to contend with only after it appeared on those pages.

In June 1977, after my graduation, I once again followed her footsteps, this time into the *Times*, and also became a copy person — running copy, getting sandwiches, and working nights. If it was the last thing she wanted, she was the last to let me know. She took me shopping for two weeks before my first day and charged everything to her accounts. She made me wear soft shoes and she was helpful in pointing out the maniacs and the geniuses and she edited my first story. And when it didn't get published, she told me that "not all good stories make it" and to get on with another right away.

The newsroom of the greatest newspaper in the world is a vast box of sound and motion. When I started, there were still huge machines spilling out yards of yellow and white copy by the second, all of which had to be separated and delivered to the various desks as quickly as possible. Now most of it comes in directly by computer and everyone can read it as he wishes.

The summer of 1977 brought the deaths of Guy Lombardo and Elvis Presley. It was also the summer of the blackout, and to me it was the best of all times. I was twenty-one, and on that incredible night when the lights first flickered and then went out in New York, I saw reporters and the best editors in journalism come in on foot and on bicycle without being called. I dashed for the metropolitan desk, grabbed a phone, and sat there where I knew the action would be good, and I stayed until late into the next morning, taking dictation from reporters around the city, one of whom witnessed open-heart surgery performed in the semilight and with a manual oxygen pump, and I knew what my father meant when he got quiet about the *New York Times*. It is a place worth every ounce of respect it commands. It is called the newspaper of record for good reason; the effort made daily, literally line by line, to be correct is as stunning as it is endless. Mistakes slip by, but they are the exception. The power of the paper is remarkable. The controversy it causes turns those who have worked there into perpetual defenders of the place. Even as a copy kid, I found myself in arguments at parties about the validity of a story, about the politics of the paper, about specific reporters. I was very proud to be working there. For even my first stories, the ease with which an interview was granted was astonishing. My father, having been there for thirty-five happy years, had developed an absolutely reverential glow when the subject was the *Times*. He told me I would love it, and I did. I loved seeing the reporters come and go daily; I loved the news; I loved the finished product, sometimes put together and ripped apart four times during one night because of breaking stories. On the night of the blackout, and against substantial odds, we put out a paper because we knew how.

My father carried my sister's stories around with him as they were published, and on the evening of my first, he walked me up to the club, saying that he wanted to buy me a drink. My father drank only beer and drank only two, at most, each day. When we got there he pulled the story out of his back pocket and said to the man next to him, "That's my kid."

In February of the following year, my father's illness became acute.

I was working at night. I never got home before four in the morning and so woke at eleven A.M. Margaret was living in the city, and Allene was working during the day. My father and I had a pact not to tell my mother of his inactivity during the day. Mostly, he would read. He patiently waited for me to get up late in the morning and make his breakfast. I would then spend the day with him, feed him a late lunch, and go to work for the 7:15 P.M. to 2:45 A.M. shift. Late in the afternoon, he would get into bed, where he would stay and from where, when my mother came home from teaching at the preschool, he would tell her he was tired and had just lain down.

He was a marvelous liar. She never believed he would lie about anything, so in a situation like this, he had her convinced. She never saw the shock of his inability. She never saw his delusions. He was afraid to scare her off. She was in love with her independence, and so was he.

My mother could not take care of my father in his illness. All her life, her greatest effort would be to "make nice" — not because she believed in it, but because she didn't, and that made it hard and therefore worthwhile. When she did anything for anyone, she expected something in return. She wasn't ruthless. She was what she considered practical. Hit her, she'd hit you right back. Compliment her, she'd thank you; need something, and she'd do it, for which you'd do something as thanks. She had a very hard time with his illness, because cancer to her meant the person wasn't going to get well, so she couldn't help, she couldn't do anything that would bring improvement, and she therefore thought she could do nothing. She liked to see an improvement; she liked to leave her mark.

One day I called the hematologist and insisted that my father was failing. I was disgusted with my inability to change anything I put my hands on. I couldn't save him, and I was sworn not to tell.

A few days after my conversation with the doctor, followed by another in which I reiterated my belief about his deteriorating health, the hospital called. My father and I had agreed he'd go. My mother said we were both being overcautious, but I prevailed. The hospital said that it had a bed. My father had answered the phone and replied that he didn't need it. He told me several hours later, when I was bringing him his breakfast. He asked what all this was about a hospital. He told me he was fine. He was wrong. For the first time, he was wrong, and he was confused. I didn't understand just how confused. I had never seen anyone be confused, especially not someone I loved — especially not him. He was so organized, always so precise. All of a sudden he was unsure of the day, of how to dress, of what to say to the person who had called about the hospital bed.

I called back and reserved the bed. I looked at the calendar and counted the three weeks since I had noticed a distinct change in his health. Three weeks of this private collusion. But at that moment, on the phone, I was all alone. He was confused and unwilling to go along with any plan.

I took him into the shower. It was the first time, in memory, that I had seen him naked. I was crying. I was embarrassed, and as the water streamed down us, me dressed, him not, I wept and sobbed, but he was too weak to be in there alone. I was determined that he would go to the hospital this time, but that I would have him back home again with me.

My mother wasn't home. It was Saturday, at noon. She was rarely home these days — gone early in the morning to teach school, home late in the evening after the various classes she attended. On weekends it was always one thing or another — a gallery, a museum, the library. I drove my father to the hospital. When an attendant wheeled a chair up to the car, my father gently pulled his wallet from his back pocket and handed it to me. He was giving up. He was never the same after that moment. He didn't answer any of the questions they asked in Admitting.

I tried to sign him in as best I could. His wallet was like his filing cabinets, which were like his sock drawers. Two months earlier, my mother had threatened to leave him if he didn't clean out his file cabinets. He had always been a reporter; he always took notes. Notebooks, cocktail napkins, matchbooks, everything was saved. A pack rat of quotations and impressions. I was amazed, one day, to find the files empty.

He winked at me and took me to his sock drawer. There, eight inches deep, were the notebooks, the licorice he hoarded, the napkins, the ticket stubs. The socks were with his shirts. My mother had not ironed in fifteen years, or done laundry. He was safe. And Eva, who did the ironing, was totally charmed by him and was on his side.

While I was sitting in Admitting, weeding through his wallet, my mother rushed in, coat flying around her, purse clanging. She said she had been with Janet Kaplan at the museum. She looked embarrassed and she apologized to me. She realized in an instant, when I stopped her from speaking, that there had been something she had missed: that he was dying, and that she was the last to know.

During the last five days of his life, my father's mind led him back to the Rockaways, where he had fished and scouted for crabs in the brine. He was toxic from the levels of calcium in his blood and he was on strong pain medication. He believed that it was 1914 and his father, then a carpenter, was planing the tall red doors for a church on the West Side of Manhattan.

One day while I was feeding him lunch in the hospital, my father looked up at me and pulled his thinning wrists against the makeshift restraints that lashed him to the sides of the bed.

He accused me of putting him in the hospital. He wanted to go back to the beach, he said, and I was keeping him there. He was furious. There was nothing worse. He never got angry. He had been the most patient of men and had the softest face, a lather of wrinkles. Seeing it strained with confusion and anger frightened and hurt me.

He had lived with his cancer of the bone marrow for five years, in terrible pain, and at the very end of his life, his mind started to wander; the disease was taking his greatest strength.

He started bellowing at me. I was shocked and terrified. I had never seen him drunk. I had not seen him weep but once, when his favorite cat fell out of a tree. I had never seen him shake with rage. His mind, leaving him, even allowing him to be in short pants, on the beach, happy with his father, unnerved me. I could not understand why he would want to live in the past. Yes, he had had a youth that he recounted in detail for those who would listen, in snatches, as children do. But the present was his family, his reading, his pride in us, his joy, his hopes. Dammit, we were the present, and I couldn't understand what was so horrible that he would rather be in the Rockaways. I thought it was the worst part of the cancer I had yet to see. Probably it was the first time in five years that he didn't feel excruciating pain. We were told that the cancer had caused a huge calcium overload in his system, particularly in his brain, and that that was the cause of the confusion.

My mother scolded him later for scaring me. He had cleared up a little and he was ashamed and hurt that he had upset me. It was the last time we spoke as father and daughter. The next day, he was back at the shore.

On the fifth night of his hospitalization, the doctor phoned and told my mother that we should come. He said my father was going to die soon. My mother called me at work and arranged for me and Margaret to meet and join her. We stood in a pavilion in New York Hospital beside a man who was in a coma. I kept telling myself that it "isn't Daddy." I couldn't stand to think that he was in pain, and I wanted to believe that it was just his body there, not he. In my head, I kept singing, "My Father," a song by Judy Collins. The lyrics tell of the promises of a father and the hopes he has for his children. Over and over in my head, like a torture.

My mother wanted to be alone with him. "I feel so guilty," she kept saying. I couldn't understand guilt, I felt no guilt. I couldn't understand how she knew what she was feeling. That song was running riot in my head, and guilt was the last thing I was feeling.

It was Margaret who finally told them to let him go if he started to die. Earlier in the night he had, and the hospital had saved him and kept him alive until we got there, and I stood and listened to my mother agree to let him go and all I wanted to do was tear down the hall and fight him back to life.

The doctor told us to go home, not to wait around. It was very late, and the doctor was quite sure that he would die but thought we should leave. I remember my mother just gathering up her stuff and obeying and telling us to do the same.

The three of us went to Margaret's apartment. At 1:10 in the morning, the phone rang and I began beating the walls with my fists. It was less than two hours after we had left the hospital. Margaret said thank you into the phone and I got up from the bed where my mother and I were going to sleep together and I pounded the walls in the hall, and my sister hung up the phone and said, "Come on, we should be together now," and my mother said, "No, let her go," and I pounded the walls over and over and I knew I never again wanted to feel such relentless anger and such monumental grief. I did not want him to die.

With all the pain he had felt, with all the changes in his

life that his cancer had demanded — he had lost more than half a foot in height, had slowed in walking — I wanted him to live and fight it. I wanted him with me.

The next day my mother and I packed many of his things. We had the energy of the sleepless. She discovered the sock drawer and she wept. I tried on his cap from the Navy. Dull and slow and then with moments of glee, we worked and discovered and remembered and wept. My sister stayed in her apartment and made arrangements, renting a hall, calling his friends.

I went out for a run. When I came back, my mother called downstairs, "Douglas, from South Africa, called. He's in Paris."

Three and a half years. I have graduated from college. My father has just died. We had written. I had sent pictures. He sent a friend to see me. But he had never called before.

"He's going to Rio."

I had sent sonnets. He had written back, saying that I couldn't spell.

"He'll call back. I told him your father died. He's coming to New York."

What timing. When I walked into the hotel room, it was for me as if I'd never left.

"Look, Eddie," he said, without saying hello. "Legs, child. Look, Eddie, she has legs," he said, pointing to mine. Of course Eddie was with him. I wasn't even surprised. They went everywhere together.

"Hi, Eddie," I said, trying to defuse Douglas' mania.

"I never knew she did. All she ever wore was T-shirts, Eddie." To me, "Little darling, you've got legs." Then, "Eddie, out with you just now."

Douglas sat in the back of the Quaker Meeting Hall, where we had the memorial service. The place was packed. None of us actively practices any religion, and this building downtown was big and old and a perfect place for the long-time friends to tell stories about James Pilkington Roach. Bob Daley read telexes they had exchanged when my father was his editor and he was a young man, in Spain, determined that the *New York Times* would print column-length pieces on bullfighting. His father, Arthur, was the first sportswriter to win a Pulitzer. He was one of my father's closest friends. They used to play a game called sardines when Arthur was married and my father was not and my father would descend on the newlyweds in Riverdale at all hours. The Daleys always said that they met the nicest young women at those hours. The game was like hide-and-seek, and one night my father hid on the window ledge, outside, two stories up. A police officer came by and asked what he was doing.

"Playing a game" was the reply from the tall redhead.

"Play it inside," snapped the cop.

These were the things we heard. Joe Nichols told of their long friendship, of how my father was so young when he started writing for the *New York World* that his father would drive him to assignments. Jim Tuite, my father's successor as sports editor at the *Times*, spoke, and Pat O'Brien introduced the speakers and gave a speech of his own.

I was surprised that Janet Kaplan didn't show up; I had expected to meet her. My mother didn't seem to notice, and my sister just rolled her eyes when I mentioned it and said, "Oh, Marion, forget it, will you?"

To prepare me for the memorial service, the King of Scotland took me for a helicopter ride over Manhattan. We lunged at the Statue of Liberty and dipped down over Central Park. It was a warm day in March. It may have been the wrong time to go dancing, but it was, in fact, the wrong time to grieve. Three months later, it hit, and I grieved and cried and began the lifetime project of missing my father and loving the small things. But for five days in March, I showed Douglas New York, and we ate and, yes, we danced.

Chapter 5

THAT JUNE my mother and I went to the Belmont Stakes to see Steve Cauthen ride to a Triple Crown. We cried in each other's arms as he pushed that big horse over the finish and we said in unison, "He did it for Daddy."

In the summer of 1978 came the newspaper strike, which lasted eighty-eight days. It was fun at first. I went to the Adirondacks and splashed in the falls where I had splashed as a student. I sat in a diner reading the upstate news and learned that the Pope was dead, but I missed that big newspaper every day, like that big horse at the finish.

During the strike Margaret was being wooed by *Women's Sports* magazine in California to move out there and be its editor. She took the job, and we went out together to look the place over. Margaret moved, and my mother and I remained living happily together in the house in Douglaston.

That fall, I was very surprised to have my mother tell me that she was glad to be going through menopause. She said she was glad to be getting over "the bother." Some bother. Thanks, Ma. You said it was a wonder.

She said that she'd had some fears, but now that it was actually happening, she was glad. She didn't seem glad. To me, she seemed preoccupied. And she seemed slightly forgetful — little things: her keys, a lunch appointment. In a woman as aggressive as she, the change was a relief. She was taking herself less seriously. She was laughing at herself. I was laughing with her.

I read about menopause. I read about it behind my mother's back. I was afraid that there would be a black side to all this giddiness. I read about the pituitary gland and about hormones, about breasts and cancer and depression, hot flashes and occasional confusion. Depression, I learned, can cause listlessness and confusion. That was all I needed to know. So we improvised. I made extra sets of keys; I reminded her about bills; I watered the plants. We still had our seven cats and a happy, if slightly confused, household. Every now and then an article would run in the paper about memory. Most were about the early onset of senility. I would scan them, but by and large I ignored them. I was interested in menopause.

And I was interested in where my mother went sometimes; occasionally she came home quite late. She had started using her memory problems as a defense. When I asked her where she was on a Saturday night after she had been gone all day, she would laugh and say she "didn't remember." I joked about it with her.

One Saturday, I went into the city to visit some galleries. In the afternoon, I developed such terrible menstrual cramps and such frightening dizziness that I called work and said I wouldn't be in. I drove home very slowly, feeling worse by the minute. When I got there, I was in severe pain and was bleeding heavily. I could tell that I must have been white in the face, and when I walked in and my mother ran to me at the door and asked what was wrong, I replied only that I wanted her to help me upstairs.

She stood over me in the bed and again asked what was wrong. I explained. Then she asked where I had been, and

I told her I'd been in SoHo when the trouble started. Had I "seen anything strange there?" she wanted to know.

I was a bit annoyed at the question. I just wanted to sleep. I said no, and she asked once more, and then asked if I was sure. It was as though she wanted to tell me something but really wanted me to guess.

That was so like her. My mother didn't have a philosophy of life, really. She reacted to incidents. She did not completely accept the responsibility of her own actions and could be like a child when confronted with something that she herself had done wrong. She would rather be found out than admit to anything.

When she asked me whether I had seen anything that I thought could have made me sick, I wondered whether she believed in voodoo or felt that if she did something wrong that was unrelated to me, in some way I would be hurt, not just emotionally, but physically.

That incident was among several that I found myself recalling; they kept coming back, that day and the keys and the forgetfulness, and I would wonder if I was missing something, if something was really wrong with her, and then I would dismiss all the incidents as unrelated and therefore matters that could not hurt us. I always thought of her and me together; she was right about that.

After the strike was over, I went back to work as a copy girl at the *Times*. My mother's fiftieth birthday came up early in November, and I had decided to throw a surprise party. The strike had given me the time I needed to plan it.

One hundred and sixty people were invited. Everyone in the neighborhood volunteered to bring food. There were hams and turkey, casseroles and punches, salads and desserts, and the house was festooned and splendid. I had picked out all her favorite records, only to find that most of the people wanted disco. When Lette, a woman who at this time had begun a good friendship with my mother, asked about the music, I proudly told her all about the jazz records we had. She seemed uninterested. She said she'd bring her record of "Saturday Night Fever." I laughed, but everyone wanted to dance. I got my way at the beginning of the party, though. I put on "Wait 'Til You See Her," sung by Joe Mooney, just as my mother was walking in the door.

The few close female friends my mother had were like lightning all night, helping, cooking, making everyone relaxed. It was strange, because not everyone seemed terribly comfortable at first. I hadn't had very much contact with some of the people in years — hellos at the tennis courts, questions about their daughters; not much more. It was so odd to me. Some people seemed surprised to be invited.

"We don't see that much of your mother anymore," one woman said. "She seems to have, you know, another life."

No, I didn't know. But I let it pass. For her friends like Lisa, Lette, Elaine, Norma, and several others, the party was great fun.

It had always seemed to me that most of the other women my mother knew were jealous of her. And for good reason. She was a beautiful woman and she knew it and she enjoyed knowing it. She was a blonde in the moonlight and a redhead at sunset. She looked great as both. She was well educated, devoted, articulate, and well read, and she had remained a magical athlete.

I had let a lot of things pass that people said to me over the years. Jealousy was for other people. My mother was never envious. If she wanted something she lacked, she would set her mind to it and acquire it. It seemed to me as simple as that.

When my mother entered her surprise party, she was duly surprised. She playfully berated me for doing such a thing to her. She was beaming, though; she looked beautiful and elegant. Everyone danced late into the night.

I composed a toast: "To the person whom I love and respect more than anyone in the world."

I remember it, because I remember wondering whether it should be "who" or "whom," and I knew that my mother would correct my grammar, even then.

The elation of the evening was soon forgotten. I had hoped it would linger, that it would make her happy for a long time. It didn't. She literally forgot it. A week later and then a week after that, I mentioned the party and she looked startled. She said something like "Oh, yes, uh-huh," as though she were appeasing me. She seemed distracted and unhappy. Every once in a while, that winter, she was even more forgetful; she would ask me the date in a concerned way, as though she had no idea. She seemed very concerned about something, preoccupied.

Then my mother began speaking in vague terms about wanting less responsibility. She had stopped cooking. She was eating yogurt nearly every night for dinner. She had stopped talking about having her fur coat shortened.

In the spring of 1979, I was promoted to a clerk, working during the day, on the metropolitan desk. "Working during the day" at a newspaper means coming in at eleven in the morning and leaving some time after seven. It was a great job. I worked for Sydney Schanberg, who had won a Pulitzer for his writings on Cambodia. I admired him tremendously. Mostly the job was phone work: taking news from people over the phone, trying to get the good stories into the paper, sharing the "nut" calls with the other clerks and sometimes with others.

One evening, I called my mother at home. "Hey, Ma," I said into the phone, "check this out." I had just heard an end to her favorite maxim. "Live each day as if it were your last, for one of these days you may be right." We both laughed like hell.

The clerks' favorite calls were the bizarre ones we received daily, by the hundreds. We would signal each other to listen in.

"Hello. Oh really? You say you just killed your wife? Uh-huh. Hey, guys, I've got a hot one on line seven. Uh-huh. Really killed her, huh? Are you sure?"

One afternoon that spring I got a call from my gynecologist. "It's Myriam Selinger."

I loved Myriam. She had guts. She got to the point. "There's something wrong with your mother."

One of the clerks leaned across the desk and asked, "Got a hot one?" but I shook my head and saw a look of real concern on her face.

Myriam continued. "I told her several things to do to prepare for an office procedure. She wrote them down at the time. She did none of them. She doesn't remember my telling her, and, Marion, she has disappeared from my office."

My mother had been given a mild intravenous sedative for the office procedure. She was told to lie down for an hour. She was gone when the nurse checked on her. It was not serious, Myriam explained. She was dressed; she was certainly aware and not at all sedated by this point. But Myriam thought I should know.

Disappeared. My mother doesn't disappear.

"Has your mother told you about her condition?" Myriam asked.

She hadn't. But I didn't say anything. We kept, I thought, nothing from each other. And if there was a secret, I'd be damned if I'd admit that I didn't know it.

"She has a precancerous condition and I have advised a hysterectomy," said Myriam.

Cancer. The very word made my teeth ache.

"I'll call you back," I said.

Myriam's office is located across from the Tavern on the Green. I had a feeling my mother would have parked the car there. I called. She had been there, sitting on a bench. "Yes," said the attendant, "for a long time, maybe an hour. Then a man came and picked her up."

I screamed into the phone, "That doesn't make sense; nobody picked her up. My father is dead. That doesn't make sense."

(I remember telling a cab driver, on my way to see my father one of the last times, that I was afraid he was going to die before I got there. Why do we speak the truth, in panic, to strangers?)

"Look, lady, she's not here."

Click.

I left work. She was in Douglaston when I got there, home in bed. She said she had driven herself home and what was I doing there and what was all the commotion; she was tired and she didn't know why in the world I was worried. But, by the way, she wasn't going to Dr. Selinger anymore, because she didn't understand what she was talking about.

We both forgot about it. She found another gynecologist she said she liked, and I didn't pry. They were talking about a hysterectomy, but nothing was definite.

That summer we had a burglar alarm installed. I began to get accustomed to my mother's forgetting the key and also to her setting off the alarm in the morning when she went out the back door to get the paper. I had reached the point where I could go from a deep sleep to running down the stairs, key in hand, in about thirty-five seconds. After forty-five seconds, the alarm would call the police and neighbors. One morning I didn't make it, and the police came, guns drawn.

I explained the alarm to my mother — how to turn it off and where we hid the key — but invariably I would find her standing in the downstairs hall, with the alarm sounding, the contents of her purse spilled on the shelf under the hall mirror, searching for the key.

Once at three A.M. the alarm rang, blaring through the house. A real break-in, I thought. Several seconds later, it stopped. Mommy, I thought. She must have been letting in a cat. And she must have remembered how to turn it off. Good for her. I rolled over.

Several minutes later she was standing in my room with a handful of tangled colored wires. She had set off the alarm and, not remembering how to turn the key, had gone to the large control box and ripped the wires from their connections. I put my arms around her shoulders, which were quivering. Then I took the clump of wires from her and directed her back to bed. She was very upset, and dismayed, but quiet.

Later, I phoned Margaret in California and told her about the burglar alarm, and as we began to discuss it, I was sorry I had called. I didn't really want to analyze it. Margaret did. I thought my mother was having a string of bad luck, and I saw no reason to dwell on it. It must have sounded very strange — first wanting to tell Margaret and then denying that anything was wrong.

I had made two wonderful female friends at the *New York Times*. That brought my total up to three. Tracy, my friend in college, had moved to New York the year after graduation, living first with us in Douglaston and then in Manhattan. We remained very close, but once she moved out of the house, we saw much less of each other.

Marianne and Mary worked as copy girls, and it was the differences between the three of us that made us such good friends. Marianne showed up her first day of work in jeans, a T-shirt, and sandals. Mary arrived in the latest from Paris, including high heels and white anklets. Marianne had grown up in a conservative Greek family in Astoria, Queens, and had put herself through Barnard College. She got her job at the *Times* by being talented and then by bombarding the head of personnel with amusing greeting cards. Mary was the daughter of a leading heart specialist in Paris and an exquisite mother who was an art dealer.

Each had an apartment of her own. Mary was urging me to share one with her, and one day that fall our conversation became somewhat strained. I heard a tone of disapproval at my "still living" with my mother. I just didn't think I was "that old" that I needed to be on my own.

And I adored my mother, and living there was easy. She was leaving me more and more alone. As I was telling that to Mary, I was struck by my own observation — that my mother was talking less, withdrawing — and then I tried to shelve it. She was indeed leaving me alone. She was canceling dates with me and becoming uninterested in my life. Perhaps it was time for a change. So I planned to stay in Manhattan for two months, apartment-sitting.

I enjoyed it. One night in November, just after my mother's fifty-first birthday, I called home and got no answer. The next day I called her school early. She wasn't in yet. I left a message in broken Spanish. She didn't call back. On Wednesday I called the school again.

"She's not in," I was told.

"Do you know where she is?"

"No. She hasn't been in all week."

"This is her daughter."

"Where is she?" the voice asked.

The tables were turning.

I was at work. I called home. No answer. I called again.

Someone answered. A groan, and the phone was slammed down, but not in its cradle.

A groan. Why a groan? Whose groan? I called back. Busy. Busy. Busy.

Knuckles to teeth; be rational; there's a reason. My mind went blank, wanting to defer, forget, cleanse, have it go away. Go away. But I had to do something. Panic. The dry heaves of the heart. My heart was beating; my eyes were working. I was dressed and ready to go, but go where? The editor sitting next to me didn't even look up but asked me to page someone in the newsroom on the loudspeaker on my desk. I did, and when I heard my voice over the microphone, sounding just like the way it always sounded, I thought I was going crazy. I sounded too calm. I put down the mike, and the man tilted his head and gave me a questioning look. I got up from my chair. I felt the same way I had when my mother called me at ten-thirty one night in March 1978 and told me to meet my sister and get to the hospital to see my father because the hospital said this was it. That night I had put down the phone and walked through the newsroom and into the elevator and through the composing room, where my father had worked for so many years, and went into the sports department, where he had been editor for sixteen years, and found my sister, and in front of all those people, thinking all the time that I was just going to tell her to take her things and come with me, and get her alone so as not to have her embarrass herself when she fell apart, I had become hysterical, sobbing and shaking as soon as I saw her.

Oh, God, I thought to myself, this time I have to get up again in this same damn room with all these typewriters and someone yelling "Copy!" and I have to go home. Alone. Margaret is in California and I cannot call her and tell her that there is someone groaning into the phone in Douglaston. I cannot call her until I know what is wrong. Until I see for myself, alone, what has happened to my mother.

"I have to go home," I said to Sydney Schanberg. He must have seen something in my face, God knows what, and he told me to go.

I didn't call anyone. I knew she hadn't been murdered. I knew. I had once interviewed a woman who had shot and killed her husband. He had beaten her every day of their marriage. They were married for thirty years. She told me that the night she killed him, she knew as he was beating her that this time was different; she was the expert and she knew that this time he was going to kill her. This time I was an expert. On what, though? On fear? On anticipating disaster?

I ran into Mary as I was leaving the *Times*, and when she asked where I was going, I said, "Home," and circled through the revolving door. I got a train to Douglaston and started to walk from the station. A friend passed in his car and stopped after a few feet when he realized it was I. I asked him how his day was. I didn't explain my being there, but I accepted his offer of a ride. I didn't ask him to come into the house with me. The panic had pared down my actions to what was essential. When he pulled up in front of the house, I had my keys in my hand. No fumbling. Automatic. I thanked him for the ride and told him to hang around his phone, if he could, when he came home again at the end of the day.

The air inside the house was musty. The windows downstairs were all closed. It was hot and still and silent. I went upstairs and found my mother in bed, eyes open, not moving. As I approached the bed, she shifted her head, but showed no recognition. She didn't speak. She smelled. Her hair was dirty and oily and matted and there was an empty vodka bottle in the trash basket and one in an open underwear drawer. The phone was off the hook, lying on the floor. I asked my mother to sit up. She refused. She wouldn't speak. I lifted her arms so that I could pull her up and put her in the shower. She snapped her arms back and lay there, staring at the ceiling.

I called Dr. Prutting in the city and described what I saw.

He said it might be a stroke; it might be the alcohol; it might be that something had happened to upset her and she had decided to get drunk. It might be these memory problems I had once mentioned to him on the phone. Was I ready to think of that?

Was I ready? Was I ready? Was there something he had been thinking and not saying or that I was not hearing? Was I ready? Was I ready for what I was seeing there in her bedroom? You bet I wasn't. I stood over my mother with the phone in my hand. Dr. Prutting told me to ask her certain questions, to check her pulse. After ten minutes of various attempts that elicited what appeared to be a stubborn refusal by my mother to answer, and no symptoms of a recognizable medical problem, I hung up and went into my room and called my sister. I next called another friend in California whom I loved dearly and who, not realizing my dismay, started to tell me that he had just been denied a hearing in his divorce case. It was then that I started to sob. I cried and cried to him how awful that was.

"It's bad, honey, but not that bad," he said.

"Marion!" came a shout from the other room. "Marion, where are you? What is it?"

Pat, pat, pat, bare feet on a wooden floor, on the hall carpet, on the stone floor, pat, pat, pat, into my bedroom, and there she stood, my mother, who ten minutes ago didn't know who I was. She was standing in the doorway of my bedroom, hair almost wet with filth, pajamas misbuttoned, arms out. I put down the phone.

"Why are you crying? God, tell me what it is?" she demanded.

I hoped I was losing my mind. In the course of the past hour she had seemed comatose and then just angry and stubborn, and now she was up, talking, making sense, recognizing me. Recovered.

She was rocking me in her arms, and I sobbed and sobbed,

and she said, "Oh, my God, it's me, isn't it? My God, I've done this to you, I have. Marion, there's something wrong with me, I know there is, but don't you cry. I promise that whatever it is, it won't happen again. I promise."

Two weeks later she disappeared from the house for four days. She had no idea where she went. I still have no idea where she went. I only know that when she came back, she was an emotional and physical wreck and that she was ready, she said, to find out what was going on in her brain.

Chapter 6

WHEN I WAS A CHILD we went to Dr. Schneider. He had a red brick house with an office right in the front, and as I sat in my undershirt with the thin straps, he would tell me to look at the blue bird on the windowsill and then stick me with a hypodermic needle.

It didn't last long.

"Don't start!" I snapped at him one day when I was about six. He had just gotten to the part about the blue bird.

My mother always said "Don't start" when she saw a fight brewing between my sister and me, when the dog started to whine at the door and it was raining, or when Grandpa got the cards out to give us a poker lesson.

"Just don't start," I said to the doctor.

My mother wheeled around and looked at me sitting on the examining table. I remember the look. It wasn't shock.

After Dr. Schneider, there was a lady down the block whose specialty was splinters and then there was the gentle and kind care of a neighborhood doctor across the street who kept her hair very short and who was forever sending me for blood tests, which almost invariably made me back off my concocted symptoms.

By the time I was sixteen, we had progressed to Dr. Prutting. My father had the great luck to take me to his Park Avenue office the first time. As we shared a cab up Madison Avenue, I was jotting notes. My father leaned over, looking pleased. A short story, perhaps.

"No," I replied, "stores. Look at all these stores. Names of stores," I said, looking down at the pad. It was my first ride up Madison Avenue, or at least the first when I was of an age to pay attention to clothes.

And so it was to the Park Avenue doctor that I went with my mother's memory problems. I say I went, because at first I went alone to discuss her problems. After I had seen him I would call Margaret and she would call him and they would talk and she and I would talk and I figured we all were talking about — thinking about — the same thing, and that that was good.

I watered down the incident of my finding her in the bed. I said that I had been "hysterical" and that she was fine after she got out of bed. Dr. Prutting seemed to go along with the new version. He said, "Your mother never was very good with liquor."

It shocked me. My mother had been a drinker as long as I knew her. As a child I remember seeing her drunk after parties, late at night, never during the day. I remember hearing her in the kitchen getting a drink; I wasn't ever really upset by it. Margaret never drinks. She never has. She says she had a sloe gin fizz once, but that's it.

I remember single incidents of my mother's drinking and it was these which filled my head like mud as Dr. Prutting spoke. He was speaking of a "history of drinking." I was thinking of separate incidents, each one of which had been forgiven. Incidents. Single happenings. He was talking about a pattern, a lifetime.

I was thinking of incidents of forgetfulness. I wanted to know how to stop them. He was talking about a pattern, about "progressive deterioration" of her memory. I was telling him about the in-between times, her clarity, her conversation. I just wanted to know what to do if one of them happened again. He started listing them, counting them off on his long fingers: the keys, the burglar alarm, my finding her in bed, the disappearances. Then he said the word "disease." He said she might have a disease. And I stopped listening.

My mother had begun to lie about her memory. She would say of a phone number, with a smile, "Oh, I can't think of it now. I'll go look it up." And then I would find her, minutes later, staring at the floor, on the verge of tears.

Dr. Prutting had known my mother for many years. It was he to whom my mother had taken Margaret for those sessions, nearly twenty years before. At this point he was in his seventies and active. I went back again and we sat in his office, where there hung two pictures of my father.

Dr. Prutting, suspicious and brooding, would draw his slender fingers down the sides of his cheeks, as if to extend an already elongated face. He tried a new tack. He said he thought that my mother was depressed. She was depressed. He used words like "fascinated" and "tranfixed" and "curious," referring to his interest in her depression. He said he was fascinated by my mother's desire to do less and less. In all the years he had known her, he said with a smile, he had never found her "dull." No, she was not dull. We talked about her beauty and her tennis, her grace and her wit. He nodded and smiled, and we agreed. I said that she certainly was an "interesting" person, and he said she was "flamboyant." Maybe, he suggested, this was part of the pattern of her extreme nature. Maybe this was just the way she was going to be now.

He got me. He had laid a trap so big and so powerful and so painful that all of a sudden I was the one insisting that there was something wrong with her, that this was not just a pattern of behavior. If there was something wrong, it certainly could be cured; it could not be allowed to go on and on like this.

But it was not a disease that could be cured.

No, I thought again to myself later, she's not dull. Not after the business with the cats, the disappearances, the confusion. Not to me. Not in the middle of the night, naked in the kitchen, or in my room asking me if it was Saturday. Not after all those incidents, which were surprisingly beginning to look like a pattern.

Almost overnight I became furious, confused, and unwilling to bend. I reported her every behavior change to Dr. Prutting. A thin guilt was developing; I was acting badly toward her, and I wanted to justify my anger, my confusion, my stubborn refusal to allow her to be naked in the kitchen at three in the morning. She was the bull in the china shop, and I was the detective, the spy in the house.

After he saw her himself, Dr. Prutting thought that she might have an allergy to alcohol. Fine, I thought; that's it. The treatment? She was advised not to drink. She stopped — we did it together. I figured we had it licked. Some people recommended a chiropractor and a nutritionist, which my mother and I figured could not hurt. We also tried long walks and ginseng tea.

Her memory didn't improve. But her denial did. She would resent the slightest suggestion that she might have forgotten something. What had at first been charming, almost eccentric, in a women who had never been "ditsy" was now nasty and frightening and provoked great defensiveness in both of us. What had been a sifting through her purse — even dumping the contents — as she looked for her keys became her throwing the full purse on the floor and storming out of the house. What was a silent look of forgetfulness became a face gripped in torment, as her fingers pulled at her hair, her voice uttered low and terrifying moans — all over, perhaps, a phone number.

I started coming home later and later. I had purchased a car and I would go away on the weekends, to the Adirondacks, mostly. I was visiting old friends and sometimes boyfriends, kindling flames that were never meant to be. I couldn't be honest about my sudden dropping in on people, my need to get away from my mother, and I wouldn't justify my inconsistent visits. But I didn't want to be there with her. I was working until ten P.M. at the *Times* and did everything I could to stay out late — five, six in the morning. One night, after the rounds of Upper West Side bars and a long sweep through a cavernous dance palace on the East Side, I ended up sitting on a grimy stoop on Forty-fourth Street and Ninth Avenue with a young lawyer. Why there, I have no idea. It wasn't safe and it wasn't sane, but it was becoming typical, and there we sat until dawn, he in pinstripes and cuffs and I in a yellow wrap dress, with two glasses and a bottle of champagne.

Throughout the fall of 1979, I called my sister constantly, asking her advice, alerting her to changes, complaining about the hostility that was building up between my mother and me; Allene resented being watched and I resented having to watch. Margaret searched through magazines, books, and the minds of doctors.

When we first unearthed some details, what we found, more often than not, were articles about memory loss and its various causes and how they were related to senility. I looked up the definition of "senile." The dictionary listed it as "pertaining to, characteristic of, or proceeding from old age." My mother was now fifty-one years old. She was not old. She could not be senile.

I remembered a man who had died recently in Douglaston. He had had terrible cancer and been in great pain. At the end of his life, in the hospital, he retreated into his great sailing days. When people visited him, he would tell them how to rig the spinnaker and would then take them along on a cruise to Essex, Connecticut, or to Montauk. But he had a disease; he'd been in pain. My mother wasn't in pain; therefore, she didn't have a disease.

I kept thinking that my mother might be kidding. Maybe she wanted me to take over running the house. Maybe she just wanted to relax. Hell, I thought, she certainly was going out of her way to get what she wanted.

I thought I was covering it well. I thought it wasn't really bothering me. When it did, I thought that I was overreacting. Then one night a friend of mine at the *Times* found me alone, leaning against a wall and crying. It was as if I had come out of a dream to find him standing there, with his hands on my shoulders. He asked what was wrong and I spent thirty minutes rambling on about my mother — about how I didn't know, I just didn't know what was happening, why she sounded so strange on the phone, why she frequently seemed surprised by her own surroundings, as if she had just appeared there, to me an image in a zoom lens, to her an image awakened in some strange place. And why she was growing hostile toward me.

Mary said that my mother sounded "jealous and angry" when she answered the phone and that she would hang up abruptly without taking a message. At the same time, my mother developed a curious routine of spending time, wrench in hand, under the sink in the kitchen, saying she was going to "find that drip, find it," when there was none.

Dr. Prutting had set the stage. He got me to believe that something was really — medically — wrong. It was painful for both of us. But then, despite our desire to find a cure, he got nowhere. I felt terribly angry. He had led me to this awful state of awareness, and as I began to feel abandoned, I became more enraged. He had gotten me to think that something was wrong, and then he had no answers. I couldn't go back to that unblissful state of ignorance, and we couldn't move forward. It was dreadful. I was angry with him and embarrassed that I had ever told him such personal and ugly details about my mother. In fact, I was learning my first lesson about how little is known about diseases of the mind. And I was learning — although I didn't realize it then — slowly learning, to refuse to let things be. My mother always told me to cut my losses. But this was one I wasn't going to cut, and I wanted real help. I wanted Dr. Prutting to find something so that we could cure it.

Margaret told me to keep looking. I didn't know what it was I was looking for, because actually I was looking only for it to stop, not to know what was wrong.

Margaret became quite stern with me. I kept calling her in California and telling her the details of the visits to Dr. Prutting. Finally, she said she had heard enough and insisted that our mother be taken to a neurologist. I found one and it was Margaret who spoke with him initially. She must have thought that I would have wavered, that I would have played down the circumstances to a stranger.

My mother and I went to see the neurologist. It was just three weeks since my mother had had the cats put to sleep, just a year after she had begun losing her keys, a year and a half since my father died. Several of my mother's friends spoke with me beforehand about how I had no right to put my mother through such an "embarrassing" procedure as a neurological workup. It annoyed me. They weren't living with the problem and I didn't think that an hour with a doctor would be in any way as embarrassing to her as losing her keys and forgetting the date. I didn't think that her friends were as embarrassed to answer her occasional questions as I was to find her swaying over me in the middle of the night with the expression of fear and confusion that she had when looking at me.

It was her look, her awareness of her forgetfulness, that was the worst thing for me to witness. It was when I saw her fear, her anguish, her clutching my pocketbook and saying it was hers and then putting it down, staring at it, realizing that it wasn't hers, that I was smack up against having to think that something was wrong and that she knew it too. She knew better than anyone that something was wrong, and it tortured her. For all the times she asked a question, there must have been thousands of times a day when she was too ashamed to ask. Knowing her as I do, I know that she was ashamed. And then she'd be fine. She'd function perfectly well. She'd be absolutely confident and secure and happy and on her way, and I would shake the image of her dismay from my mind. She couldn't deal with her anguish, and I wasn't going to.

But it would come back. It was like a little wound on my knuckle: move it, it opens up; leave it alone and I knock it and it opens up. And many times it was her friends who opened it for me.

What I once thought was love and respect from some women her age, and just tolerance from others, gave way to stunning hypocrisy. All of a sudden they were busy. All of a sudden my beautiful, athletic, witty mother wasn't such an attraction at dinners, for tennis, for bowling, for sailing, for an evening swim.

I began to realize that those who truly cared for her found something they feared, some failing on her part that could be theirs, something that many of them didn't want to know about. It was at this time that the group of friends — both close and occasional — began to dwindle. Then, when she needed them most.

And when I needed them, too. My mother needed her friends, and I thought I needed an adult to talk to, to defer to, if necessary. But for the most part they weren't around. And I wasn't ready to ask for help.

What they did volunteer was gossip. Almost as though she were always out of earshot — already dead — people began to sidle up to me and tell me the most horrendous stories about her. People who had known her for twenty years would tell me about an occasion when she had been "real drunk" or "real loud." Someone suggested that she had been having an affair "for years."

So what? That was all I felt. Just so what? Their gossip was no help, and help was what I so desperately needed.

That afternoon when we went to see the neurologist, I heard my first memory test — that afternoon while I looked up First Avenue at the people staring through their windshields, that day when the answers came easily only as we crept back into the past.

The doctor diagnosed her as having a slight memory problem. No surprise. He said that we should "monitor" the problem for a while. I left there with a soft sense of dread.

I got to work thirty minutes late, and my small boss (not Schanberg) yelled at me. I was standing by the metropolitan desk and he started in on "I'm going to have your ass," half-kiddingly, half-not, and I felt my face redden.

"You know where I've been?" I shouted. "You want to know?"

People were staring. It was 3:35 in the afternoon in the newsroom of the largest paper in the world, and the place was packed. "You want to know where the hell I've been? I've been watching my mother prove that she's losing her mind. Leave me alone." And I went to my desk.

Margaret came home right after Christmas. I could see that she was worried; she was questioning my mother's abilities. After a few days she asked me what I really thought of Mommy's behavior. I was embarrassed. I was just watching, but not in any way allowing myself to think that something was really wrong. It was behavior, I said. Margaret gave me a critical look. She said that it was her opinion that our mother was very depressed and that it might be related to the menopause. My sister took my mother to the gynecologist, the one my mother had chosen and had been seeing on her own. The doctor said that he had found a precancerous condition and had suggested a hysterectomy but that my mother had said she would "let him know." Margaret immediately scheduled it. Both Margaret and I believed that the operation would help.

It didn't.

After the hysterectomy, Margaret extended her vacation and took our mother to the follow-up visits. To my surprise, Margaret dressed the wound. She explained that our mother wasn't up to taking care of it herself. She suggested that the scar, the reminder of the surgery, might be too traumatic. It was very odd to see Margaret care for her.

It never occurred to me that my mother would need any help. Not her, not my mother. And if she needed it, she wouldn't ask. Not my mother, not the one who always told me to cut my losses and burn my bridges and live each day as if it were my last. Not her.

Margaret doesn't believe that every day may be the last. Margaret believes in building things. She believes in careful change. Margaret never abandons something she can patch. I am sure that if something is leaking, it is sinking.

Again, I was receiving clear lessons about the differences between my sister and me, and this time it was more than just Margaret's using the blunt scissors as a child and my trying to use a sharp wit. It was the ability to mend, the ability to see that someone needed help.

I was very aware of my mother's state when she came home from the hospital: she was depressed and confused. But I was certain that it had to do with the procedure and that the "change of life" must be extremely depressing and possibly confusing.

Margaret returned to California. I read more about the secretion and absorption of hormones. I went to interview a woman who had written about menopause, ostensibly to talk about another issue, but I got her on the subject of her book, and we spent four hours together, discussing my mother's menopause.

By the spring of 1980, four months after the hysterectomy, my mother and I had joined a gym in Manhattan, where we both worked out with weights and took steam baths. Occasionally she stood me up. She spent at least one night a week in the city. She said she was staying at the apartment of her friend Janet Kaplan. I asked her why I hadn't been able to find Janet's address in the Rolodex when I was planning the surprise party, and my mother said it was because she remembered it; she didn't need to write it down.

"Funny," I said, "you don't seem to remember much else."

She shot me a vicious look.

She began a regular pattern of standing me up at the gym, which was four blocks from the *Times*, and I began to get slightly resentful. I always looked forward to seeing her and to the competition: the weights, our weight, sit-ups, leg-lifts.

I liked living in the big old house with stained-glass windows. I liked the privacy. My mother left at 6:15 in the morning. When we lived together it was not on top of one another. She seemed to enjoy it, too.

The other thing my mother still enjoyed was her work. She continued to drive in early and tell me the stories of the home visits and the new theories of teaching preschoolers to read and count. She seemed to have no doubt about her work; she was confident and was continually coming up with better ways to teach the children to read, to count. She'd try out some of the theories on me as she revised the

Montessori method to fit her needs. She was very comfortable with the idea of teaching and enjoyed the curiosity of children.

Then, late in the spring of 1980, six months after that first neurological exam, while we monitored my mother's condition, her memory problems seemed to take a rest. She was luxuriating — we both were — on a plateau of her semiconfusion. Both of us felt we could compensate for it. She had five sets of keys and there were several hidden around the house. She had megavitamins and early nights and Canadian Air Force exercises and more of my company. She didn't seem to be getting any worse.

We went to the ballet. We went to museum openings. We went to a Picasso exhibit one morning. In the car she thanked me for going with her. That was surprising. I had been looking forward to going. She asked me if I wouldn't mind driving. She hated my driving. She always told me I drove too fast. I reminded her of that. She said she didn't really mind it.

While we were looking at a display of his cubism, she turned to me and said in a whisper, "I'm sorry, but, well, I don't like these."

This was a woman who never apologized and almost never whispered.

"What's wrong with you?" I asked, impatiently. "What's all this humility?" If she was going to be humble, she was leaving me out on a limb. I wasn't going to take humble, not from the woman who told me always, every time, to enter a room as if I were the most beautiful woman there and that that action alone would ensure that I was.

"What do you mean?" I insisted. Now people were staring. "You don't have to like this stuff. Have an opinion, dammit. I hate it. I think it's garbage." We left the museum.

In the car she turned to me and put her hand on my arm — this woman who never touched anyone; who once, when

I asked her to hug my father in front of me because I had never seen her do it, told me to mind my own business. "You really ought to learn to control your temper," she said sweetly. "I never realized you were such a hothead." I almost drove into a building.

A few months later, in the fall of 1980, my sister announced that she and her boyfriend, Gregory, were giving up their little house outside San Francisco, that she was going to leave the magazine, and that they were moving to New York. Margaret was to return to the copy desk of the *New York Times*. I thought it was nice. She was coming home in two ways.

At first, everyone seemed very happy to be together. And it was grand to have a man in the house again. We used Greg to move things around, and I really loved having him there. But I was kidding myself. In the early days any change seemed good. Any new action was a distraction.

Within a week things were bleak. Margaret and Greg thought that they were going to stay in the house for two months or so and then move into a place of their own. Margaret knew from our phone conversations that I wasn't happy. She said that she would come home, "whip us into shape" (a favorite expression in our family), and then everything would be fine. It was more than fine with me.

Although Margaret and I had kept in very close touch, she was shocked by my mother's condition and by the condition of the house. Despite my unhappiness, I was clinging to the parental image of my mother; there were certain things that, despite the illness, I thought must somehow have been getting done. But I was wrong. Bills that I thought had been paid were shoved into the pockets of her Ethan Allen desk. The roof leaked. A heating system that was costing us more than $6500 a year produced little heat and almost no hot water. The basement flooded continually. I was exhausted and depressed, and so was Allene.

I had, unconsciously almost, started calling her Allene by this time. It seemed impossible to say "Mommy, do you have your keys. Mommy, you stood me up for lunch again. Mommy, you asked me that already." Mommy wasn't the same old Mommy she used to be, so she was Allene.

Several weeks after my sister and Greg moved in and it became apparent that they were going to stay, I took a sublet in Manhattan in a building across from a funeral parlor on Amsterdam Avenue. The house was just not big enough for all the personalities involved, and Margaret and Greg, I figured, deserved their privacy. Also, I wanted to try living in the city again. My sister threw herself into work on the house — changing the oil heating system to gas, fixing the roof and the basement. I threw myself into getting to know my new neighborhood and living a new life.

At the end of February I went to Switzerland with Mercedes, a friend from Douglaston who was a great skier. When I ski, I tend to throw my body around, exhausting myself but making little progress down the hill. My mother used to say proudly that she was the only person who ever graduated from the University of Colorado and never skied. Maybe there is a connection with my inability.

Mercedes and I went to Verbier, a pocket of warmth tucked into the mountains. We had some hysteria over a young masseur who spoke no English to me while he looked down at all my aching muscles sans skiwear and spoke the King's English to Mercedes when he asked her for her room number.

When I returned to New York I went to Douglaston for the night. I walked into the house with my tan, my ski bag in hand, ski boots on a rack, also in hand, and suitcase in tow.

My mother answered the door. She was holding one of the surviving cats. She said, "How was work, dear?" turned on her slipper, and went upstairs.

Greg later confided that he thought my mother was very "weird."

While in Switzerland I had met a young man named André. "If you are ever in New York . . ." Three weeks later he called and asked why I hadn't answered his cable. "What cable?" I screamed into the phone, my vacation flashing in front of me.

"Is it all right?" asked André through the crackles of the terrible overseas connection.

"I'm fine. Is that what you asked, André? Okay, then, bye." I put down the phone with a sense of dread. I didn't know him at all and we had just skied together and had a few beers and we barely spoke each other's language. What I hadn't understood on the phone was that he was coming immediately. He'd called from the airport.

I farmed him out to all of my friends. He and I had lunch with my mother. She came to meet me at my apartment. My sister drove her in, and when I opened the door my sister was shaking her head and saying, "Marion, Mommy. Marion lives here."

When Allene came in she saw a picture of herself and my father. "Who lives here?" she asked.

"Who are you?" she asked André when she noticed him. "Who are you?" she asked him repeatedly over lunch at the Tavern on the Green. Returning to the scene of the crime. I should have known better, but she loved the place.

"How do you know my daughter?"

"Who are you?" "How do you know my daughter?" and "Who are you?" She never stopped. His English was barely passable. Her French was nonexistent. And I was so nervous that all I did was order food, only to have Allene realize that she had left her wallet somewhere. Not a great lunch.

Margaret began an active campaign of research into memory disorders. I was disinclined to join her. I hadn't seen anything in my previous, although limited, research that led me to think that my mother had a serious disorder. Also, since I had moved into the city I had begun a very active life, going out frequently with Mary, Marianne, and Tracy to bars and parties, and dating a little.

My three closest male friends were, however, old pals from Douglaston. Skip is as subtle as a nod in every gesture and handsome in a timeless and sophisticated way. He speaks as carefully as Daisy Buchanan, whom Gatsby described as having a voice that's "full of money."

Scott almost swaggers with youthful enthusiasm. And he is enormously attractive. He is clever and almost impish in his ability to provoke thought and reaction.

Jimmy is the king of nicknames; he has dozens, as he does personalities. The strongest of his traits is his consistent protectiveness of me.

Although I saw Scott more than any of them — because he would stay in my apartment more nights than not — I remained close to all three. I had a hard time making new friends, something I thought no one would understand, so I stayed away from parties where I might not know most of the guests. I was feeling very unsure and hesitant, especially when asked about my family. I ran into an old friend, Todd, who pointed that out to me.

He was studying at MIT when he got back in touch after several years of silence. He was having a show of his paintings downtown at the Ronald Feldman gallery and invited me to come. I took my mother. She and I went first through some of our favorite old haunts in SoHo. We drifted into the gallery and I saw Todd. He was doing research on the brain and mind at MIT and at this time was doing paintings — simply put — of the activities of the brain. All I saw, when we walked in, were huge, colorful images of the brain, almost flowing over the walls. The elongated and classically beautiful renditions of neurons spread across the tall, wide walls made the viewer feel he or she was inside a head. I didn't understand most of Todd's theories, but it was a stunning moment. I looked at my mother, standing in this deep tall room with white walls and my friend's images, and I heard his voice coming through a video monitor, talking about the "moment of intuition," and his voice, in person, explaining about the right side of the brain being art and the left being science, just at the moment that my mother asked me once, and then repeated, "What day is it?"

My mother became fascinated with the video monitor and moved away from us. "Her brain," I said to him, as he gave me a tilt of his head, "her brain. They think there's something wrong with her brain."

"Who thinks?"

I didn't explain. I felt surrounded and hot. I let him lead me around and explain a magnificent structure on the floor called a "Cerebreactor," which he had designed, combining the workings of the spinal column and the brain with the image of a nuclear reactor.

When my mother and I left, I took her to a little Chinese dumpling house and held her hands across the table and said, "What day is it?" She looked startled. "What day is it, Mom?" She was right when she answered that it was Saturday. I went on — What time was it? Where were we? — the imitation brain expert that I was. She became very angry when I began each question. Several times she crinkled the edges of her eyes and gave me a harsh look. But she always gave an answer, though most were wrong. I decided that she was confused. I was unfair, of course. I wanted her to know exactly which blocks we were between and what Todd's last name was and things that might have been difficult for anyone, and sometimes her anger was justified.

When I stopped and concentrated on my food, she put

down her chopsticks and looked at me, not with anger, not with spite, but with honest wonder, and asked, "Marion, what day is it?"

Todd refused to play armchair neurologist. He told me to discuss my mother with a doctor. I had.

Margaret clipped things and left them on my desk. I would scan them and throw them out. Most mentioned senility — my buzz word — which I felt justified my throwing them out. She wasn't senile. She wasn't old enough. I would tell Margaret that I was reading Todd's textbooks when I wasn't. I told her he was looking into it at MIT when I hadn't even asked him to.

One of the newspaper clips my sister left for me was on Alzheimer's disease. There was a woman at the *Times* whose father had it, Margaret managed to find out, and she had asked her all about it. The words "senility," "senile," and "aging" ran throughout the story, and I would have tossed it out, except that something nagged at me. The victim mentioned in the article was young, and the first symptoms were simple — lost keys, forgotten phone numbers — things too familiar to ignore, to forget.

I had heard of Alzheimer's disease, but I knew little about it. I knew that Rita Hayworth had it. One of my father's doctors had told me that Margaret Mitchell and Charles de Gaulle had had multiple myeloma, the type of cancer my father had, and I remember thinking that I was name-dropping in some ghoulish way when I explained to people what he had.

I had read something about Rita Hayworth's daughter and her mother's illness, and I felt very sorry for both of them, because I knew that many people would start calling it "Rita Hayworth's disease." There were so many very beautiful reasons and ways to remember her other than by some frightful disease of the mind.

I learned a lot from that one article, but there was a lot

I didn't learn. I didn't know that the handbook written several years ago for families on how to cope with a victim is called *The 36-Hour Day*, a reference to the emotional and physical overtime put in by the family and caretakers. I didn't know that the disease ravages the brain so severely that today it is known to be this country's fourth leading killer. I didn't know that there are close to three million known victims in this country and the possibility of there being many, many more. I didn't know that what may look to someone like madness is, in fact, an organic brain disorder that begins with forgetfulness and causes a progressive — and relentless — loss of intellectual and physical functioning. I did not know that it is, to date, irreversible, without cure and without any treatment except sedation. I didn't know that the doctors do not know what causes it or whether the disease can be passed from one generation to the next.

Alzheimer's disease was first described in 1907 by Alois Alzheimer. A patient of his, a fifty-five-year-old woman, had displayed "progressive jealousy" and had died following the onset of severe dementia, medically defined as a profound loss of memory, intellectual functioning, and the ability to take care of social and bodily needs. An autopsy revealed two abnormalities in the patient's brain, which we can define in terms of present knowledge. The first was the presence of neuritic (or senile) plaque, a spherical formation that consists mostly of degenerating brain cells. The second abnormality was something called neurofibrillary tangles, or snarlings of the neurofilaments, which are structural components of cells and are involved in various of their functions. These tangles appeared predominantly in the cerebral cortex and, in particularly large concentrations, in the hippocampus, the part of the brain thought to be associated with short-term memory.

The behavioral manifestations described by Dr. Alzheimer

were not new. In 1838, Dr. Jean Etienne Dominique Esquirol, an eminent French physician, had described *démence sénile* as an illness that results in a loss of short-term memory, drive, and will power, and one that comes on gradually and may be accompanied by emotional disturbances. He described it as a condition that afflicted people over sixty-five. Dr. Alzheimer concerned himself with what happened when a similar condition occurred in people under sixty-five. It became known as "presenile dementia." At this point, it was not clear to Alzheimer or other researchers that the two conditions — senile dementia and presenile dementia — were, in fact, the same thing.

Virtually no research was done on dementia during the fifty years after Dr. Alzheimer's discoveries. Then, in the 1960s, three English scientists, Dr. Bernard E. Tomlinson, Dr. Garry Blessed, and Sir Martin Roth, followed fifty demented patients who were over sixty-five through the end of their lives. After their deaths, autopsies were performed. Comparisons were made with the brain matter of twenty-eight nondemented, age-matched adults who died during the same period.

More than half of the demented brains were found to have pathological changes indicative of Alzheimer's disease. The scientists concluded that in most cases senile dementia and presenile dementia were the same disease: Alzheimer's. Most researchers estimate that 75 percent of dementia patients suffer from Alzheimer's disease.

I learned these facts from the newspaper and from a few medical magazines we found. I casually asked the people in the science department of the *Times* about the disease. They turned over some journals to us. I had started calling my mother's condition madness, but slowly I was learning that it had another name, a proper name.

But I held out. The word "dementia" bothered me. Demented. To be demented, don't you have to look demented?

Maybe her eyes had to lose their look of perfect conviction. And then, what about hardening of the arteries? No connection, I was told. Everywhere I looked, no connection. But senile. Whenever I saw the words "senile" and "senility" I remembered the part of the definition that referred to the characteristics of old age, and that released me.

As I write this, my mother is fifty-six years old. She thinks she's fifty-five. "I'm the speed limit," she said to me. "Just cruising at the speed limit."

Chapter 7

AT THE BEGINNING of that summer of 1981, I left the sublet on Amsterdam Avenue and moved into my own apartment. Finally, my own furniture, my own clutter, my own pictures on the wall. There were high ceilings and a fireplace and a bedroom just inches bigger than my bed. Tracy and Scott helped me move on the hottest day of the year. We rolled over the Fifty-ninth Street Bridge with no rearview mirror in the huge rented truck, and we split a case of beer as we set me up in my new home.

Toward the middle of the summer Margaret and I decided that what Mommy needed was a little trip. The great remedy in our family — travel. Just get away for a little while and see something new and, well, maybe things will be different.

We decided that we would accept the kind offer of Red and Phyllis Smith to visit at the end of August. Although I knew that Allene needed a little trip, what I didn't realize at the time was that my sister needed a little break.

My mother and father had been to Martha's Vineyard to visit the Smiths several times. My father had told me about the beaches and the fresh seafood; he and Red had walked along the wharf and had clams on paper plates. I needed to see the Smiths. I wanted to be with old friends. I wanted to be with someone my father's age, like Red, to remind me of my father. I wanted to be with my father. I was desperate for his company. My father never swore. My mother told me that she heard him swear only once — and that was at the television, right after Watergate, when Nixon was making a speech of guarded reassurance. My father looked at the screen and said, "Bullshit." He had voted for Nixon and he felt terribly let down. I wanted to see how my father would react — if he could be calm — in the climate of my mother's illness.

Margaret, who was going to stay behind, brought Mommy to the airport. Since her trip to Egypt, my mother had been through Europe by herself, and after my father died, she went alone to China. We were confident that this trip to the Vineyard would be good therapy. My sister and I also had some hope that she would be better — different, somehow — after the trip. Inside the Marine Air Terminal it was humid and hot and still. My sister looked exhausted.

On the plane my mother asked me, "Where are we going? Do we have tickets home? When are we coming back? Why are we going away?" Over and over again. I thought she didn't trust me, didn't think I was capable of making the proper arrangements. I reminded her that I had traveled quite a bit. She looked at me as if I were speaking in non sequiturs. I looked back at her. "Remember me?" I asked. "I am perfectly capable of getting us there, you know."

"Where?" she asked.

I gave her a book, but she didn't look at it. As we flew over Block Island, where I had been sailing at the beginning of the summer, I started describing the cliffs and the freshwater ponds. She asked, "When are we going home?" I reminded her about the Smiths and their dog with the French name. She asked, "Where are we going?" After we were picked up at the airport, she asked where we were.

When we reached the house and unpacked, I noticed that every outfit, every section of her suitcase, was labeled in large, distinct print. Her vitamins were in a plastic box with the days of the week pasted over the sections. All this was Margaret's doing. I stared at the print on the labels and it became terribly, horribly clear that, for the first time in my life, my mother was not capable of doing something completely by herself.

I should have realized it sooner. My sister, in the ten months since she had moved home, had practically restructured the entire house and household, and that included my mother's life. I had seen the roof, the basement, the gas burner, but I had been avoiding the change in my mother. But looking at the labels, I could no longer ignore it. More than the house had changed. And Margaret's role was enormous.

My mother spent the weekend in a state of high agitation. She could not sit still. She followed me into every room, asking me again and again when we were leaving, whether we had tickets home. She slept soundly and deeply. She ate like an animal. She reached for things that were not offered to her. She tapped her feet incessantly. I would grab her knee, under the table, holding her leg down, and softly but firmly ask her not to do it. Once, after two days of this, she looked up at me and said, "You're hurting me." I looked down and realized that my nails were pressing into her flesh. I had done it so much and so often that she had two little blue spots on either side of her knee. I was mortified. But she kept it up. I would explain to her that the tapping interrupted conversation. She would say, "Oh, I'm sorry, I didn't realize," and look at the other people and seem genuinely aware, and I would think, Now she understands. Oh good, that's all I had to say. Maybe she's got a hearing problem and a nervous tick. Maybe it will be all right. And then it would start again, barely half a minute after she had seemed so aware. Tap, tap, tap, quick hard beats on the wooden floor.

Phyllis brought out a coffee cake the second morning and put it down more than arm's length from my mother. My mother reached out, grabbed at the box, ripped off a hunk of the cake, and stuffed it into her mouth. I was horrified and scared. But I didn't know what to do or say. Red and Phyllis were perfect. We had been friends for many years. Red had written my father's obituary. Phyllis has the kindest eyes and the gentlest nature I have ever met. The Smiths were an unbeatable pair.

Red would lie on his stomach, in the evening of that weekend, and sneak puffs on my cigarettes. He wasn't supposed to smoke, ever, and I certainly shouldn't have allowed him, but I couldn't resist him. We all went to the beach. He brought his boomerang, and we tried to make it return. He — over seventy, a hat the shape of an upside-down tulip squashed on his head — was better than I. Then he told me to swim.

I was nervous about leaving my mother with them. I was afraid of what she would say. He looked me in the eye, and then up and down, and at my shoulders. "Go on. Your father told me you were a great swimmer. Let me see," he said.

I went out about twenty yards, freestyle. I looked up. Red waved his hand in the air, parallel to the coast. I turned and swam. After a while I relaxed into the rhythm. I looked up, he nodded, and they got up, the three of them, and walked down the beach. They called to me to meet them at the house. I watched as Red, Phyllis, and my mother slowly walked along the beach. Red could not manage the stairs up, and he used a level exit farther down. But he had the mind of the greatest living sportswriter. He remembered every story about Toots Shor and boxers and foot racers, some stories that were sixty years old. And he took requests.

My mother didn't know what day it was. And he had twenty-four years on her. I was twenty-four.

Later that night Red just talked at dinner and my mother listened. She would join in on the obscure dates and names of people on the train to the Derby, and she would smile to think that she was helping him along. Then she would turn to me and ask if we had tickets home.

I cried when we left. I cried to be alone with her again. I cried because I thought I would never see Red again. I was right. I cried because I was scared and because I did not understand. As the plane took off, she asked, "Why are we leaving?"

Margaret met us at the Marine Air Terminal. I was not expecting her, but I was relieved to see her, to be able to tell her about the weekend. My mother slipped into the ladies' room. I knew that something was wrong. I knew because my sister was there and because I saw her look at me as if to weigh my feelings, judge my strength, assess my reaction to having been with my mother.

"It's Alzheimer's disease," she said. "I spoke with the doctor this morning."

I was carrying Truman Capote's *Other Voices, Other Rooms*. I know I was because of the way the book looks today. I looked down at the copy in my hand and then I looked at my sister. She let out a high, pained cry and reached up to cup my shoulders with her small, soft hands.

I turned away and started beating the walls with my book. Margaret put her head in her hands and cried, convulsing her delicate shoulders in tremendous, terrifying waves. I continued to hit the wall and stride around the reception room of the terminal. Around and around, shrieking, bellowing, really, hitting the walls, slapping them with the book, circling my sister, who was hunched over and sobbing.

A man came over. With his arms held out like a forklift, he shuffled from one to the other of us, a two-step of confusion, making his silent offer of help. I looked at him. I must have shown my fury. I waved him away and hit the wall again. My sister never looked up. God knows, people must have thought there was a plane crash.

My mother emerged from the ladies' room. "Where are we?" she asked.

Margaret had gone alone to get the diagnosis while my mother and I were on Martha's Vineyard. The doctor had started by saying to her, "Your mother is not going to die."

We thought that the words were offered as comfort, as reassurance. We were wrong. The words were, in fact, preparing us for something quite different, for something with no quick before the dead, with no speed but my mother's agitation.

The doctor told Margaret that to understand our mother's behavior, each of us had to imagine herself a woman contemplating losing her mind. He said that the mind will not tolerate this conclusion, and the result is the denial, the questions, the constant questions, which are an appeal for some confirming sign that she is not losing her mind. But she cannot retain the answers, and she cannot remember that she just asked the question.

Following the diagnosis, we looked everywhere for more information, for help. We became pack rats of ideas. There was no listing in the telephone book, no entry in the encyclopedia. And we already knew what the dictionary said about senility. It said nothing about Alzheimer's disease.

The idea of senility haunted me. My mother was not old. At this stage she was still alarmingly beautiful, and sometimes composed. For several months we dug up nothing. We just watched.

Chapter 8

ROMANCE, for a while, was the only thing that mattered to me. Not simply the act, but the pursuit, the promise of the dance of it, the look across the room, the gesture. I realized (not too far into what can only be likened to physical pandemonium) that it was because only then I did not have to think about my mother.

That may sound too easy, but it isn't. It happens. It is something that can take a great deal of plotting and planning, or none. And it's exciting.

The recklessness was spreading. By now, it moved into my friendships. I made dozens of new friends instead of cultivating old ones. When the new ones became older ones, I would avoid them. I was working my relationships in a manner the reverse of the way my mother's memory was failing; she could not retain anything new, but eventually, after enough hammering, the new became the old and it was retained. If she heard something often enough, somehow she retained it. Somehow, after three months, she would pick up a name, and it would go into her memory, which was like a broken record just before the skip. What day is it? What time is it? How's Gregory? What day is it?

What time is it? Previously she had just looked at Greg and asked his name, over and over and over.

My sister, on the other hand, was cultivating her old friendships while taking care of my mother and living with Greg. She was working hard on her relationship with Greg — which was obviously strained, in the climate of my mother's illness — and she had a few close friends.

I, on the other hand, formed casual acquaintanceships, and saw more of the people who cared less for me, in order to avoid all serious conversation. I really did not want anyone to know how things were with my mother; I did not want to see the panic — which I expected — in anyone's eyes.

My mother could still be quite good company. She could play tennis and bowl and she liked to go for walks. She was repetitive, and that was annoying, but she was able to discuss the past. She had lovely stories about her youth and her marriage, her trips to China, Egypt, and Europe. She wasn't getting lost and she certainly wasn't dangerous. She was confused. She was also, happily, less aware of it. She was less tortured by it and no longer seemed depressed or anxious about her memory.

But I was taking it very badly. I was hurt and felt unhappy all the time. When we were together I was short-tempered and unable to allow her to enjoy a long walk completely. I would try to get her to stop asking the same questions over and over, which was impossible. I overreacted, I suppose, but at the time there was no talking to me about it. I hated it and I was hurt.

With Mary, my French friend at the *Times*, I tried to live a combination remake of *Breakfast at Tiffany's, How to Marry a Millionaire,* and *The Lost Weekend.* A nice triple feature, we figured. A girl's got to eat, we rationalized, and nothing bad ever does happen at Tiffany's or Bendel's, I found out, and champagne and somewhat slipshod morality was better, because it was easier, than a meaningful relationship.

I met a man in a delicatessen. I should say I met a tie in a delicatessen. I spoke, you see, first to the tie. I recognized it as one from that vast range of Wasp yacht clubs. I was in black cashmere, weaving through the deli at two A.M., looking for milk, after a dinner party given by Mary. "I know you," I said to the tie. Thank goodness there was a hopelessly nice man attached to it. The man paid off my cab driver, who was waiting outside, walked me around a bit, and sent me home, where I knocked myself unconscious on my bedroom door. Things were getting bleak. The combination of the cashmere and the contusion on my forehead made me look like Mike Hammer's secretary.

I called Nicky, my loyal, faithful, sweet friend, Nicholas Patrick Madigan. Nicky had taken up the space in my life that was created when I moved to my new apartment and saw less of Scott. The apartment was much smaller and did not afford us the luxury of room for two.

It was now five in the morning, and Nicky lived on Second Avenue and some street in the single digits. A far cry from the Upper West Side. "I bumped my head," I groaned into the cold telephone. I had no heat.

He came up. The bump was there and it was blue and green and I explained about the dinner but didn't remember talking to the tie or how I got home. I tried to make jokes, but he wouldn't let me. Enough, he said, was enough. I thought so too.

But it didn't last long. I lied to my friends. I went out with people I didn't really like and continued one relationship in particular that was clearly not good for me. I never discussed my mother's illness with him — her confusion, my panic — because I believed, unlike Ernest Hemingway, to whom all references of this sort must bow, that the rich were very different, not ordinary people with money. This beau had a great deal of money, and I thought that my mother's disease revealed her working-class blood.

I was, I think, at the end of the rope, and what I wanted to do was get him to tie the knot. Maybe, I reasoned, if I became part of his world, mine would be unreal. I did not want to confront it. I did not want to know. His mother was beautiful, articulate, and aware. She was married to a very successful businessman. I admired their grace and her calm. I thought they would live together forever, because their money and their power insulated them from every evil.

That January, almost five months after my mother's diagnosis, following the dinner party and the contusion, I was floundering once more. I quit the dangerous relationship. I stayed home a lot and sat and wondered, and finally I started to pay attention to what Margaret was trying to teach me about the disease. I had reached a level of self-disgust that I recognized only when I sobered up and stayed home one night. After that, I just turned one night into another, and although the clarity of mind let the pain increase, the clarity of mind allowed the return of some long-mislaid self-respect.

Margaret had found an Alzheimer's group, part of a national network, with a branch in New York. She attended her first meeting. During a break, several of the people approached her and asked her if my mother knew what she had, if we had told her. We had not. We debated it every day. A spouse of a victim suggested that we do it, that knowing the truth was my mother's right. We agreed with that. But what we were afraid of was what reaction there might be. And we still considered ourselves kids — children — in need of an adult to make that sort of decision. One person suggested that if my mother knew what she had, that if she knew what lay ahead, she wouldn't want to live. It was suggested that we tell her and give her the option to kill herself.

Margaret called me after the meeting. She was obviously shaken. We decided that our situation would never get that bad, that my mother would never be so severely ill as to want to die. What we did not understand was that by the time she was that ill, she would not know that she was sick and therefore would not have the mental ability to make the choice if she wanted to.

My sister did explain to our mother what was wrong. Later that day she heard her tell someone that she had had a stroke, the same thing she had been saying for a year. There was no mention of a brain disease. There was no acceptance, later, when I asked her if she understood her problem. Maybe we had waited too long. Or maybe the denial was too strong.

Margaret took me to my first Alzheimer's meeting that January. It was on Long Island. I looked at people's name tags, searching for ethnic similarities. There were more than a hundred people there. I looked for wealth or poverty. There were the similar faces and dress of families. There were several people with vacant looks who seemed agitated.

Everyone wore a look of exhaustion. It was unavoidable. It was in every face, every matching brow, every clasped hand. I have never before or since been so struck by a similarity of purpose, a similarity of expression on the faces in a crowd; not at the racetrack when my mother and I saw Steve Cauthen ride to the Triple Crown finish, not in the newsroom of the *Times* when the Pope was shot.

One of the doctors was speaking. He used a pointer to stress the symptoms written on a blackboard. Among them were confusion, memory loss, and agitation. I knew all about those. My mother was up and down every moment. At the refrigerator, on the couch, out the back door, off for a walk in the rain with no coat. Next, the doctor pointed, loss of speech, incontinence, death.

I looked at my sister. "What the hell is this?" I asked.

"It's okay," she said, and held my hand. My sister is able to hold hands. And despite the fact that she prefers not to do so too often, my sister is able to hug me. It made me uncomfortable, but I held her hand then. I wanted to scream. But I decided that that wasn't the type of Alzheimer's disease my mother had. She had another type, and she was young, and anyway, she'd probably get cured. So I let go of my sister's hand, and Margaret must have known what I was doing, because she gave me a very stern look. I crossed my arms. Deception is great stuff. Self-deception, at the time, was the stuff of my life.

A man leaped up. He pointed to the blackboard. "She doesn't do that!" he shouted. "My wife doesn't do that." He gasped, waving his hand at the range of symptoms. "She doesn't have it, right?" He was a nonbeliever at a gospel meeting, and I felt the room begin to turn. I felt my sister's hand on mine. I felt sick to my stomach.

The doctors had seen this before. They asked the man where he had learned the diagnosis. They had heard of this doctor. They assured him that, although another opinion is always welcome, he had a good doctor and that, yes, his wife probably had Alzheimer's disease.

I stared at him. Keep standing, go on, dammit, I willed him. Think of something, get us out of this, I'm on your side. Oh, God, don't give up.

He slumped into his chair, and as I felt his hope go, mine went too.

Two weeks later I went to my second meeting of the Alzheimer's Disease and Related Disorders Association (ADRDA). This time it was in Manhattan. I took my good friend Howard, someone I had met at the *Times* and whom I had managed — despite my apparent inability to maintain relationships — to need enough to get to know. Somehow I knew I could trust him to witness my most mercurial qualities and stick by, knowing that I was hurting, not uncaring. A man got up to speak. He had been asked to describe a typical day with his wife, an Alzheimer's victim. "She gets up at nine, every day," he said softly. He doesn't want to scare us, I thought. "At nine-fifteen she has ten milligrams of Moban. We wait a while. Then we have a bath. After the nurse comes, we have breakfast. Then we walk slowly back and forth, across the living room. I walk behind her, holding her, slowly rubbing her stomach up and down, up and down, like I've been told is best. Then we go into the bathroom. That takes a long time. I continue to rub her stomach to help her bowel movements. But it can take a long time. Before noon she gets another ten milligrams of Moban. At twelve we put her in a comfortable seat. I brush her hair. I perfume her. I try to make her look as pretty as possible. Then we tie her in the chair."

As he went on to describe the strips of soft sheets he used to tie her into the chair, I stared but could barely listen.

Someone had stopped him for a question.

"Well, sure," he said, "like this, from the back, across her chest, although once I turned my back for a moment and she slipped down and was caught by her chin in the X made by the straps."

I put my head down on the table and sobbed.

Tie my mother to a chair. You want me to concentrate now on how to do it, as if I'm in the Girl Scouts and we're tying kindling? Do you really want me to pick up my head and learn how to do this?

It went on. A young doctor named Mayeux spoke. He was gentle and soft-spoken, standing there in his cardigan. Genetic, viral, back and forth. We had no reason, as family members, to believe it was genetic. The doctors, however, had no reason to believe it was viral.

Wait, wait, wait, wait, wait. Hold on here, oh no, uh-uh. No, wait, you mean to tell me I might get this? You mean to tell me you're saying that you don't know what the hell this is from and it may be whirling around in the air out there or replicating itself, vicious, swirling double helixes in my DNA? Oh, Mama. Oh, please. Oh, God. Oh, Howard.

Another speaker, this one a woman who talked about affording a nursing home. Another woman, in the audience, started heckling the speaker. "That's easy for you to say, get power of attorney. Sure, sure. My husband weighs two hundred and ten pounds and he's mean and he won't even let me near the checkbook and his kids hate him and I don't blame them and you want me to get him to give me the house?"

The speaker was calm but was getting beaten badly. Every suggestion she made was met with furious objection.

I stood up and turned to the heckler. I spoke loudly. I said, "I understand that you're angry. We're all angry, but you have to go to a lawyer. I did, we did, my sister and I." I felt Howard touch my arm, encouraging me. "It's not easy, but it's . . ." I was going to say it was necessary. I wanted to say "necessary" and finish my sentence and sit down. She interrupted. "That's easy for you. Your father helps. What do you know about being married to a sick man?"

"My father is dead and my mother is an only child. My father was an only child. Why are you doing this? Why are you making it so hard?" And I was sobbing in front of forty people, uncontrollably, heaving and crying, and I could not stop.

A young couple reached across the table. Both stretched out their hands. Howard, tears in his eyes, put his arm around me. And I sobbed and sobbed. I could not control it.

A woman at the back stood up. She said she was a doctor and that what we must all realize, as family members, was that this is an extremely painful and angering disability, that it takes more than one victim, and that we should be neither afraid nor ashamed of our sadness or our rage. I stopped crying. She was making sense. I looked up. She looked at me.

"There is nothing wrong with being sad about this, nothing wrong with grieving. It is not psychotic and not sick." She sat down.

At the end of the meeting, she came over and introduced herself. I saw Howard out of the corner of my eye. There was something very angry in his face.

The woman said — and I will never forget it — "I'm a doctor. You have severe emotional and psychological problems relating to your mother. It's not normal. You need psychiatric help. Here's my card."

I just looked at her. Hadn't she just said it was okay? I should have socked her. I thought Howard was going to. He pulled me away from her.

"Ambulance-chasing" was all he said. I have since found out that she is notorious for it, and I've decided that should our paths ever again cross, I will sock her.

Several weeks later, Margaret was in the kitchen with my mother. They were cooking, following a recipe. A step was left out and my sister noticed it and remarked to my mother that they had to add something.

"The best laid plans of mice and men always gang la glee," said my mother.

Margaret's head snapped up.

"What?"

"What?" repeated my mother.

"Gang la glee? What's gang la glee, Ma?"

"Latin."

Allene's writing began to change. Phone messages became puzzling. Letters began to transpose. Butler became Bulter, but he was somebody my mother didn't know. A friend of

Margaret's. Not a big concern, we decided, spies together, my sister and I. Throw out this piece of tragedy, hoard this one; we were deciphering a code here. Some days we were Drs. Kildare, proving that there was nothing here that a little potassium wouldn't cure, or chelation, or hope.

My mother just didn't seem very sick. She continued to look beautiful. She was repetitive and confused, and then in an instant she was conversational and completely convincing. And she was charming. We would sit on the sun porch together and listen to Pee Wee Russell and she would tell me that early in 1937 Pee Wee left the band and played only a little solo on this next song coming up, and then she'd play "Cross Patch," which was her favorite expression when anyone was angry, or "Let's Have Fun," and I'd laugh as her eyes would dance at that title and she'd jack her eyebrows up and down like the floozy she never tried to be.

In April an entry in my mother's appointment book for a tennis date was printed in the noon slot of the page. It read CLAIRGOES! in capital letters. The date was with Mrs. Claiborne, one of my mother's oldest friends.

My sister diligently checked every appointment to make sure it was not broken, that it was tennis, not bowling or lunch, so that my mother would be prepared. Every night Margaret would leave a note on my mother's bedroom floor that gave the next day's appointments. Listings were also in the date book.

One morning they were in the kitchen and my sister reminded Mommy that Mrs. Castro, a Douglaston friend, was coming over.

"Oh, no," said my mother in a regal tone. "I called her and told her not to come."

Now that presented an interesting problem. That would have meant that my mother was making a decision not to do something and that she had properly executed a cancelation. And that was fine but, even in those days, rare. Mrs. Castro showed up on schedule. My mother had begun a new habit of saying she had canceled something when she had not.

Several weeks before this my mother had gone on a date. She'd been going to a church out on Long Island with an old friend. The service was more of a friendly weekly meeting than a formal religious observance, and she seemed to enjoy it. One Sunday she came home and said a man had asked her to lunch. It sounded all right to us. She said that the friend who took her to church had explained to the man that my mother had a memory problem. She had been embarrassed at first, but then grateful. It eased the tension.

The man picked her up and brought her back a few hours later. My mother was in a rage. "He took me to a diner," she said, "and after we ate, we sat in the parking lot and he stared at his lap. Then he told me he wanted oral sex. There and then." She had demanded to be taken home.

A week later the man showed up at the door. Gregory heard him at the door and went downstairs and invited him in. Then he pinned him against the wall and raised him to his own eye level — six feet three inches off the ground. Greg had an even tone to his voice when he was furious, and he very evenly told the guy that he would break every bone, at least twice, if he ever approached my mother again.

Margaret and Gregory had become the parents of a young girl, a confused young girl — my mother. Allene had become a girl who just wanted to listen to jazz and tell you about the Commodore Records' sessions and Louis Prima and his New Orleans Gang. She didn't want me to play the piano anymore. She just wanted to slap on a record and sit back with someone to listen.

Just listen to my records, and I'll tell you everything I can remember.

The roles had become reversed. A thirty-year-old man and his twenty-seven-year-old girlfriend were parents to Allene, and I came on the weekends. If my sister and Greg were parents, then I guess I was an aunt, even though I still felt like a sister to this damaged child.

In late January, my mother decided that she wanted to go to Australia. Mother's good friend Lisa, one-time fellow Girl Scout leader and continuing tennis partner, wanted to visit her daughter Lynn, Margaret's good friend, who had moved there. Lisa and Allene had continued their friendship through all the years. Lisa, smart and direct, had been there every inch of the way; she had watched the progression of Allene's illness with growing concern and grief. But she made a monumental effort to help my mother. She took her out to lunch and to parties. She played tennis with her. My mother was very responsive to Lisa. They had "secrets," my mother told me with a smile one day. She said that she really appreciated all the attention Margaret and I gave her but she preferred to spend time with a contemporary. She had the feeling that we were watching her. Lisa never made her feel that way. I was a little hurt, but she was right. Lisa treated her as she always had. We, on the other hand, treated Allene as a child. It reminded her and us of the illness. With Lisa, she was just Allene, and they enjoyed each other's company.

It was Lisa who suggested that she take my mother to Australia. We were all aware, although no one spoke directly about it, that this would probably be my mother's last trip anywhere, and Margaret and I were determined that she go.

Margaret and I conferred with the doctor who had made the diagnosis. He said that with the proper supervision Allene would be fine and that the trip was a good idea, as was anything that perpetuated her independence. Her short-term memory was almost gone, which meant that she could not be alone in a strange place, but Lisa knew this and honestly wanted to take her.

Since we had received the diagnosis the previous August, we had been a little less frantic. We had a medical name for the condition. And we had learned what we could expect of the illness, so we adjusted as best we could.

They were to fly to Hawaii, then Australia, and on to New Zealand. Margaret made the plans, and they seemed foolproof. My sister can give a structure to anything, and she took on this project with a vengeance. She was going to see that Allene had this trip, despite the odds. My sister's theory is that you can beat the odds if you stack the deck. She bought my mother a new bag with labeled compartments and wide sections. She packed precisely. Everything was labeled in large print. The important documents were in Lisa's care.

The night before they left, Margaret found my mother sitting on the floor of her bedroom, with everything unpacked and most of the labels torn off. My mother had insisted that they pack a day early. Since then, she had unpacked the bag three times, and Margaret had had to hide it. Allene had begged to have it back in her room and had promised to leave it closed. There she was, in the middle of the night, clothes strewn around her, bottles of shampoo, a soap dish, and toothpaste surrounding her, and the torn labels stuck to her hands and in her hair. Margaret repacked everything and put a note on top of the suitcase that read DO NOT OPEN. We had learned that notes worked wonders. And we were determined that she would go.

Lisa was a small tough woman who had been self-employed ever since being divorced. She was resolute and capable. There was no question that if my mother was going anywhere, Lisa was the only person up to the task of accompanying her.

It was to be a five-week journey. Margaret planned to have

the house painted and my mother's room thoroughly cleaned during that time. And she was hoping for the time alone with Greg.

Lisa and Allene were gone three weeks when the call came. My mother had said that she was bleeding from her vagina and demanded to be taken to a hospital. There was no bleeding. The doctor told Lisa that there was some "mental problem." There was, he insisted, no blood. My mother continued to insist that she was "hemorrhaging," and it became increasingly apparent to Lisa that she was hallucinating.

When Lisa called, they were already in Hawaii. She said simply that there had been some serious problems and that they were on their way home. When they arrived in New York, Lisa looked exhausted and depressed. The experience clearly had been horrendous.

My mother was a different person. She stormed and stomped around the house the first night, telling us that the curtains in her bedroom were in flames. She stood in front of her broad bedroom windows, looking at the draperies and insisting that they were on fire. The next morning it was the toaster. There were, she said, flames shooting from the toaster. Then it was the television. She woke Margaret several times the next night, demanding that the television be removed from the room, that it was glowing.

She talked constantly about her bleeding. One minute she was having her period; the next, she was hemorrhaging. She went immediately to a doctor when she got home, and we were told that she was "hallucinating wildly."

I had been flooded with fear when the call came that they were returning, but I was completely distraught as I began to watch Allene during the first days she was home. She wore a goggle-eyed expression like a mask. There were no moments of clarity. She didn't remember being in Australia. She just wanted to take off her pants "and show you the blood." Constantly. Several of my friends came over to cheer her up. Scott, toward whom she felt very close, came to visit, and she looked at him without any recognition and then at me and told me that she was bleeding.

She didn't make any sense.

Margaret took her to Dr. Barry Reisberg, a clinical psychiatrist at New York University Medical Center. He started Allene on Mellaril, a major tranquilizer. We were tranquilizing our mother.

The idea of knocking out my mother was so very foreign to anything I had ever been prepared for that I found I could greet it only with fury. I was ashamed of us. I kept wanting to take her off the tranquilizers and check to see if the monster was still there.

It was. I was very reluctant to give her the pills, and when I visited her on Sundays I would give her much less than she was supposed to take. For eight hours she'd be fine, but the next day, when I was back in the city and Margaret was home, my mother would start hallucinating again about the draperies.

Margaret very gently asked if I was tampering with the dosage. When I said I was, she asked me not to. I know I would not have been so patient were the roles reversed. Several weeks later, I saw the result of my handiwork when I let my mother go overnight without the full dosage. I spent the night in Douglaston. The next day she was a pacing animal, eating with her hands, shrieking at the draperies, tearing around the upstairs of the house, half-dressed and mumbling about blood. My mother, the teacher, the sailor, the water-skier. My mother was being tormented by this disease.

In three and a half years my mother had gone from thinking it might be Saturday to seeing flames engulf the draperies. It was two and a half years since she had the cats put to sleep.

On the medication, she was a different person. She was repetitive but dulled. She seemed more resigned to her fate. She was much less inclined to fight about her schedule, about having to be with someone constantly, about taking a shower. But to me, that meant that she wasn't fighting the disease, either.

Instead of fighting, she developed a set of reflex responses that were wholly predictable. The answers were rapid, the words squashed together; one glob of speech that should have been five, six words started as soon as she heard the buzz word — shower, tulips, or birthday. If you asked her to take a shower, she would say in a rush, "I don't have time to shave." Every time. Sometimes I would ask her when she wasn't due for a shower, at night, just to test the reaction. Always, in a garble, the words jammed together before I got my breath, "I don't have time to shave."

By April she was very upset about her "memory loss." She had been on the Mellaril for four months. She was depressed and quiet and she looked like hell. That hit hard. She wasn't beautiful. She wasn't thin and she didn't care. There was no response in her eyes. Her walk slowed and she began to gain weight. She would eat anything in the house. The food bills doubled and doubled again. She would drink a gallon of soda, would eat a box of doughnuts, nine yogurts in a day.

When confronted with the realization of her illness, she would say, "I have no short-term memory. I can't think of that now, but I'll know that answer tomorrow." There was a shred. She still showed a little hope — that tomorrow she might remember something. But she never did.

I tried. I'd ask leading questions. "Remember going to the club this afternoon, Mom, and eating a steak?" It was dismal. She'd say yes and give something of a smile. But she was kidding herself, and I was trying to kid both of us.

Gregory moved out that spring. I didn't know about it for

several weeks. My sister and I never talked about anything but Allene. I don't think we even realized it then, but huge events would go by that we never discussed.

In May, Margaret took Allene along to Sears to purchase a lawn mower. My mother dragged her feet, pointing at things, picking things off the shelf. Margaret asked her to pay attention to the task of getting a lawn mower, and in response my mother reached out to the shelf and offered a box containing a small sprinkler and said, "Can't we use that?"

By this time my mother had been keeping a date book for two years. At first it was her own — her own writing, her notes, reminders. Slowly, other handwriting crept in — Margaret's, mine, Lisa's. Reminders. Dates. At first the book was a great help. We would ask her to take it out when she was particularly agitated. It always calmed her down. She would stare at it and flip the pages, seeing the things she had yet to do, reviewing some of the things she had done. She was usually very quiet while looking through it. It was a great comfort in the car; she would read it and I could drive. Otherwise there were the jackhammer questions, distracting and angering.

But by the beginning of the summer, my mother's date book, with its precise appointments written out, became our greatest enemy. Anything, even an event months away, became an obsession, a topic of constant, relentless repetition of one or maybe two questions. A wedding scheduled for October was a favorite. "What are we getting them for a wedding present?" she asked me over and over and over. Not when is the wedding or who is invited. She did not even use the names of the bride and groom. All she asked was "What are we getting them for a wedding present?" and I would know what she was talking about. Because I heard it constantly.

Scott came over nearly every Sunday and we would do

jigsaw puzzles and watch my mother. "Mommy-watching," we called it. Scott and Skip and I would have some beers at night before I went back to the city. We shared a lot of late Sunday nights.

Allene started going to a local church with one of three women who would call for her. But word was getting back that she talked throughout the service and disturbed people. Margaret found out that there was another Alzheimer's patient in the congregation and went to visit the woman and her husband. The woman talked constantly. The husband seemed exhausted. Margaret came home depressed and upset.

My mother needed complete supervision. She was unaware of her surroundings and ceaselessly repetitive. She was confused. Margaret and I set up a schedule for her care. Every Sunday morning I would go to Douglaston to care for her. Our housekeeper Eva, who had worked for us for twenty years, stayed over some nights, and Margaret sponsored Sharon, who was from Grenada, to stay the other nights of the week and several days. But Sundays were mine. It's funny, because as long as I can remember, Eva had been coming to the house, and yet all of a sudden she was my mother's confidante, her best friend. They would sit on the couch and talk.

After the first four or so Sundays I became resentful. I couldn't make plans to do anything for a weekend, and I couldn't make any progress with my mother. She sat and stared at the early Sunday morning television shows — disco dance shows and Abbott and Costello — and she smoked. By eleven I was hopelessly depressed. By four in the afternoon I was pacing and in tears.

My mother stares at the television as if it were playing her song; staring into space and remembering some sweet touch, a first glance, an embrace. I sit and wonder how she can have this staring look, as though she's remembering something, when she has us convinced that she cannot remember enough to be left alone. Is she transfixed by the television show or does she remember something of her own? Or does she remember nothing?

I used to try to think of nothing as a child. I remember that well. It never worked. At best, all I thought of was that I was trying to think of nothing. But it remained a good game, a good consumer of time on car trips, for years.

When my mother first got sick I used to try it on the sly, like a child whose mother tells her not to cross her eyes or they'll stick. Instead of believing it, I chanced it, and hoped my mind would go blank for a second and then snap back. Then I became terrified of it, and in my deepest moments of despair over her illness I'd think it had gone blank for a flash and I would wish I'd never tried it.

I sneak a look at my mother while we watch television together. She looks disheveled, her soft curls askew, a look of anger and confusion on her face when things happen quickly on the screen. My mother, a college graduate, a journalist, and then a teacher, used to tell me that watching television "rots the mind." Now, it's almost all she wants to do. It's her favorite pastime. Most of the time she doesn't have the sound on; she just stares at the screen.

The television on the sun porch is fifteen years old. The color comes in patches, as if someone drew outlines of a face and then cut out colored felt pieces to fit in the outlines and never quite got around to it. The pieces float separately, but they touch. Sometimes they just flip endlessly, like fruit in a slot machine. And the set is clever. Just when we're ready to heave it into the street, it comes back. It's as much a part of that house as the record player, which still has a notch for 78s. Under the player are the leather books with paper envelopes for those thick 78s, the ones with the little white squares glued on with the name Allene Zillmann.

My mother bought a big "Cleopatra" chair when we lived alone together. It is wicker, and looks like an asp — all puffed out on top — and its towers over the tallest person sitting under its rounded head. My mother sits in it and smokes, staring at the television. She hasn't smoked in thirteen years. Now she smokes and smokes. She'll smoke four packs a day if we let her. When she shifts in that damn chair, it crackles and snaps. When she leaves it to get a match, check the time, go to the bathroom, it snaps by itself over and over, abandoned like that, for an hour, I'll bet — though I've never timed it — as if it has a memory. I've gotten to the point where I think everything has a memory. We got Allene a phone with memory dialing. It can do what she can't. I resent that. It can call me at my apartment in Manhattan if she pushes the button next to my name. It remembers my number. My mother doesn't.

When we go for a walk, she complains that I walk too fast. When we go home, she wants to go out. She now goes to church very infrequently, but as soon as she gets home — or if she doesn't go, then as soon as I walk in — she wants to go to the local tennis club, where there is a brunch on Sundays. Immediately. She'll be sitting on the couch with her coat on when I arrive. Or pacing. Or watching television.

When we get there, she wants to go home. If I get her coat, she wants to stay. My friends are much better than her contemporaries. They invite us to sit with them. With only two exceptions — and they are exceptional friends — her peers rarely invite us to join them, and many times we sit alone, in a corner, and she tries to eat with her hands and I correct her and she looks at me with anger and reaches for an egg on her plate with her fingers, folds it over, and shoves it into her mouth.

And then she questions and questions me about some detail, spraying her food, dipping her filthy fingers in her water glass. We never talk about cutting our losses over these lunches, or living each day as if it were the last. We talk about table manners.

"Don't talk with your mouth full," I say.

"Why not?" she asks, egg dripping down her face.

God Almighty, I don't know what to do.

Looking back over that spring, I think of her failings. February was when she returned from Australia. March, always dreadful, was worse because I had to go there every Sunday. By April she was completely confused. By May she was worse.

Chapter 9

IN THE BEGINNING of June 1982 I began having memory problems. I would lie in bed and count back from a hundred by sevens. I would go wrong by the third subtraction. I would forget what I was doing. I would try to remember everything I had done during the past week. I would try to remember the names of my teachers, in order, from first grade. My mother could still do that.

Every Sunday morning I would go to Douglaston from homes of friends where I had been since Friday night or from the city. I had a headset player, and I would listen to Ella Fitzgerald. I would listen to the tape over and over.

I was resentful and I was scared about going every weekend, but I was afraid to speak about it. I was afraid to tell my sister how much I hated it. It wasn't that I hated seeing Allene; I hated seeing her that way. I always thought she'd be better. When I wasn't with her, I imagined her as I had known her, so seeing her ill was a shock each time. I was shrouded in the cloud of denial. I spent many Saturdays in the Hamptons with friends and I was meeting an entirely new group of people. I would always have to explain that I wouldn't be there on Sundays for a softball game of a barbeque, and I hated explaining it. I could not think of my mother as an invalid. It wasn't that simple. It was too sudden, she was too young, and my feelings were too complicated for me to accept having anyone think that I was going to care for an aging parent. But there was no way to resolve it.

On Sunday Margaret worked on the copy desk at the *Times* until eleven P.M. and I was to stay with my mother until Margaret arrived. Usually my mother and I went to the club. On one such day, as we sat in the sun, I was reading a collection of Red Smith stories. He had died five months earlier, in January. We had not told my mother, because we knew it would upset her and also because, selfishly, I did not want her to ask about it over and over. It was still too painful. I missed him very much. He was almost the last of the people who reminded me of my father. I still had Joe Nichols, and I plagued him for details whenever I saw him — details about the track, the night boat up the Hudson, the press box, my father's expressions. I lost Joe in December.

I was reading Red's book, and she grabbed it out of my hands. "Look, Red. He's dead, isn't he?" she said. I don't know how she knew.

I had another book, and since she seemed fascinated by Red's, I let her have it and I read mine and let the conversation drop. After a few minutes, I looked out of the corner of my eye and noticed that she was turning the pages rapidly, then stopping, reading, and then turning a few more. I looked more closely. The dust cover was upside down. She gazed at me and then looked back at the book.

"I like this," she said with a nod, keeping her eyes on the book. I leaned over and turned the book right side up. She looked very hurt and put down the book and put on her bathing cap and sat there, staring at the water.

I went to get a drink. I drank a lot those Sundays. It dulled my senses. It dulled me. I thought it dulled the pain, but it didn't. Depression causes listlessness and confusion. Alcohol doesn't help. Depression causes loss of memory. So does alcohol. I knew that, but I didn't believe it.

I would go back to the city at midnight and I would lie in bed and cry, without moving, just letting the tears roll down the sides of my head. I couldn't think about anything but the shock and the pain and that the next day was Monday, and that was all I could remember. I didn't pay attention to anything else. I wouldn't remember what my mother and I had done that day. Nothing got in my brain. I would forget the titles of books I was reading and I would panic.

Then I would have nightmares. Horrendous, long, intricate, colorful dreams of my mother drowning, of her being pushed out of a plane. One morning I woke happy, thinking she had died. Then, realizing my relief, I cried and hid under the covers and called in sick to work. The dream had been so very real.

The next night I dreamed that she and I were sitting in the back seat of a station wagon. I had my hands around her throat, and she was glaring into my eyes, grinning. I was pressing and twisting her neck. I was trying very hard to strangle her, turning my grip on her throat. I kneeled on the seat and leaned into her, and she kept grinning. She said, having no trouble with her wind, "I'm not going to die."

I was teetering. I was having the most sensational mood swings. It was the first year of my life that I had noticed the sway and dance of the tulips on Park Avenue. Then I was desperate when they withered. I walked by the bare nubs one day and started to cry. I noticed an Oldsmobile on the FDR Drive with the license plate LUCID and I laughed, and then I daydreamed that it smashed through the divider and ripped into the oncoming traffic. I imagined heads through the jagged glass on the windshield and rounds of confused tire marks on the pavement. My heart started to pound. I was panic-stricken.

My mother's illness was affecting my opinions on everything. I argued with people about medical care. I cried when I saw mothers and daughters together in public. I became sensitive, almost dangerously so, to confused, homeless people I saw on the street. I tried to talk with several and was always more depressed afterward. There were subtler changes, though, that showed up suddenly, sometimes on surprising subjects.

I was in a car, talking with my friend Howard about the ideals and goals of marriage, when I heard myself say that I never wanted to marry. Howard was as undone by my mother's illness as I, and we'd had a very difficult time together on the subject. He was the one to push the truth at me very often, as he did this time.

"There can be no real commitment between people," I asserted.

"You're wrong." He has a mother, a sister, and countless aunts and uncles. Well, to me, they are countless.

"You can't promise me that you're not going to die or go mad. I don't want any part of it. I'd rather be alone. I'd rather live each day as if it were my last. God knows, I could get hit by a truck tomorrow." Then I was sobbing, hysterically sobbing, thinking about what I had said, realizing that I really meant it, too, that I was scared and angry about people dying. I was sick and tired of it.

He stopped the car and grabbed me by the shoulders and began shaking me. "Live each day as if it's your last. I hate your mother for ever telling you that. It's careless and dangerous, and that part about the truck, that's a beaut. Now you really don't seem to have a commitment to anything."

We'd known each other a long time. He'd accused me before of carelessness and the inability to commit myself, and he'd been right every time. I really did believe in living each day as my last, and I never thought about the cost to other people who might want me to stick by something, to stop looking for a back door every time I agreed to do anything. "We're not talking about me," I sobbed. "It's my mother. Leave me out of this, for once, will you?"

"A lot of the crap you believe is just crap," he said, "and because she told it to you and now she's sick, you're clinging to it as if it's a drug. But the bottom line here is that you're really letting your mother's illness get to you."

It was true. And I did not want any more of it. I did not want any more grief. No more death, no more Sundays, no more questions. No more wondering about how long it was going to last and what was coming next and when my life would start again, only to realize that this was my life and how much I hated it, how much I wanted each of those days, those Sundays, to be the last — of something, but not me. My sister had it every day, but I had always thought that her distance throughout their earlier relationship kept grief at arm's length from her.

My sister had said she hated my mother, and I believed her. I had heard it all my life. And yet I was selfish with my grief and I didn't realize that, although the horror Margaret experienced watching my mother's illness progress might have been different from mine, it was just as real. It was affecting Margaret's life in ways I was just beginning to see.

She and I were sitting on a couch one Saturday. We were with my mother, watching television. A baby came on the screen.

"Oh, look, babies," I said.

"You're sick," my sister said. "Babies, great, not me, oh no. No more custodial relationships. Uh-uh. If I ever have to take care of another person, I'll scream. I'll kill myself."

My mother just stared at the television and smoked. My sister and I looked at each other and said nothing.

I understood. But she didn't mean it. My sister, the gardener, the patient listener and tireless and almighty doer for other people, was angry and there was no other place for her to vent it.

My depression grew and I developed the most remarkable stomach aches. I went to Dr. Prutting. My stomach was swollen. Everything I put in it made it hurt. Barium tests and blood tests later, he told me that I had the beginnings of an ulcer. Terrific. It was my second.

My first was when I went away to college. I was worried about my parents, worried about my father's illness, worried about being away from home for the first time.

Following the diagnosis of the second ulcer, Dr. Prutting sat me on the examining table. He put his freckled arms around me. "Marion," he said in his gentle voice, "please. I know you. I know this stomach. I know what's going on. You cannot let it take you, too. I am going to put you on certain medications and a bland diet. And I think you should see a psychiatrist."

I left the office and walked for about ten blocks. I called a friend from a phone booth. I cried and cried into the receiver. I told him about the test results, about the psychiatrist. That, he said, might not be the worst idea. "It's okay," he said. "I'll take care of you."

It wasn't what I wanted to hear, but it was just what I needed to hear. A psychiatrist and I'll take care of you, all within an hour. It was just what set off the worst emotions of fear and trembling and, thank God, some kind of self-preservation.

I didn't think I needed a psychiatrist. My problem was very specific: I needed to learn how to manage my life within the environment of my mother's illness. I needed a handbook, a guide. What I needed was to talk with other people who had Alzheimer's disease victims in their families. Other than Margaret. I didn't need to drive Margaret crazy with any more of my doubts. I didn't want to be taken care of. I wanted my mother back and I wanted back my self-respect. None of it seemed terribly hard to understand. I wanted my mother back the way she was and at the same time I was trying to give myself away to various men I met. I desperately wanted to be loved, but I didn't want to be protected, to be taken care of. I wanted to flourish in love, not to be shielded. I didn't want to be taken away from my problems; I wanted to be able to do right by my mother and to be strong. Being taken care of was the last thing I wanted. I stood in the phone booth and I stopped crying and I went to work.

On the way in the cab I thought to myself that I didn't want to be saved; I wanted to be cured. I realized that, with greater frequency, people were telling me to calm down, not to let it get to me. I was hearing it from friends, from doctors, from people I worked with. I was beginning to think that I must look and sound like a wreck, but then I saw that it was not that simple. My conversation included references to my mother and most of them were quite horrible to the uninitiated. People would ask me how my mother was, and I would tell them. But these were people who had no contact with an Alzheimer's victim. And for the most part their reaction was the same: ignore it; don't do it; she's lived her life; let her go. Cut your losses.

My mother probably would have said the same thing — about someone else. That was the trick. As many times as she had told me to live each day as my last, to give things up when they fail, I knew she'd make the exception for herself. I knew she wanted me to fight. At the time, however, I wasn't fighting. I wasn't even trying. I was grieving and I was inactive. She was losing the battle and so was I.

But when others said it — that I should cut my losses;

that she had lived her life — I always thought, At fifty-four? She's lived her whole life at fifty-four and I shouldn't react? What I had yet to learn was how to react.

Dealing with an Alzheimer's victim is an unending and sometimes thankless task. An Alzheimer's victim cannot remember that you just answered the question, that you just picked up her clothes, that you just fed her, bathed her, directed her to the bathroom. She cannot remember and so she asks and eats and makes a mess and comes careering out of the shower, soapy and half-bathed, uninterested in your frustration, unaware of your rapid impatience, of the fact that you are repeating the answer, the action, again and again and again.

It is frustrating, but I wanted to learn how to do it, and when I wanted to bitch about it, I wanted someone to listen to me.

During that long summer, my mother began to be very hostile to Margaret. My sister has a small and intricately delicate frame. She has beautiful soft small hands with broad, smooth nails. She has the largest blue eyes I have ever seen. She is asthmatic and sometimes has leveling attacks that can put her in bed for two weeks at a time, at which time her feminine and softly lit bedroom becomes a house for a breatholator and oxygen tank and tissues, the bed piled with magazines and television guides, the room filled with quiet and concern. When she becomes ill, it is frightening, because the onset is quick and the attacks virulent, and she coughs from the depths of her small lungs and looks overheated and tired. Her attacks have always frightened me because they so completely take her strength.

One morning when I arrived, I saw my mother walking behind Margaret on the stairs and I saw her watching the cadence of Margaret's careful step, and it frightened me. That morning, my mother had grabbed Margaret at the top of the stairs, and it was not clear whether my mother — who outweighs Margaret by thirty pounds and is four inches taller — was considering hurling my sister down the stairs. I had walked in right after this incident. Margaret was very upset. My mother consistently was verbally nasty to Margaret and about her. But this was the first physical demonstration of hostility. This was different. It was a Sunday. My sister was on her way to work. After she went out the door, my mother made some comment about "the warden" being gone.

We were walking back up the stairs. I was behind her. "What do you mean, warden?" I asked.

As far as I could see, my sister's care was gentle and careful and preserved my mother's dignity and was a blessing, and I could not understand any hostility from my mother.

"Warden Margaret. Do this, do that. I hate it. I want to leave."

"Leave? Leave? Where are you thinking of going? What do you mean, leave? This is your house, and Margaret lives here with you, and . . ."

We were at the top of the stairs. She grabbed me by the shoulders and started dipping us downward. I broke her grip and pushed her like a chest pass in basketball, backward into the hallway. She turned and went into her room.

I am five foot nine and weigh 135 pounds. I am taller than my mother and in pretty good shape, but she had had a solid grip on me and there was something in her eye that I had never seen before.

I ran into her room. I was in a rage such as I had never known. I grabbed her by the shoulders and started shaking her, her big shoulders firmly in my hands, her head wrenching back and forth. I was shaking the daylights out of her.

"Stop it!" I screamed. "Stop it! Leave Margaret alone. You never paid enough attention to her. She's not like us. Hit me, go on! For fuck's sake, I'll give you a decent fight. You want to throw someone down the stairs, come on, try it on me. Let's go back to the stairs. But leave Margaret alone! She's sick, she's tired."

I was still shaking her, whipping her neck back and forth, and then I let go and we stood looking at each other, and she closed her eyes and said, "Oh, God," and turned away and I stood there, looking at my palms, which were scarlet, and she went to her dresser and pushed a few pieces of loose jewelry around and then turned to me. "What day is it?" she asked.

I was beginning to come around — to give in, give up, maybe — but it was a long, slow process.

I had another dream. I was standing on the front lawn, trying to fix the broken wing on a bird that alternately became a lobster. I couldn't get it to work. My father walked out of the house. He looked around for me and came over. He was dressed in madras shorts and a hat with a band. He was obviously relaxing somewhere and I had disturbed him. He didn't look as though he minded, though. After all, it was a long time since we had seen each other.

I continued to fret about the bird-lobster. He took me aside. He said, "I have three things to tell you. First of all, don't get married. Not yet. Live like me. Second, work hard. And the third is that the situation with your mother is going to be over much sooner than you think."

"Oh, Daddy." I looked at him.

He said, "I have to go now. I'm fishing with Red."

He vanished. I woke up, and for the first time in a long time, I woke up laughing. I was accustomed to screaming, crying, and shrieking as I sat bolt upright in bed, clutching the covers, clawing the air, screaming for attention. I wasn't accustomed to waking up smiling.

I paced back and forth in front of Marty Arnold's office. Marty was the deputy editor of the *New York Times Maga-*

zine. I wanted to write a piece about a woman who had killed her husband. I had been trying for six months to get up the courage to talk to him about it. It had been rejected the year before by another editor of the magazine, but I wanted to try again. I wanted something to do.

Marty always paced. Up and down the halls with a frown. We paced together and talked. I tried to match his step, his concentration on his pacing. I tried to make conversation. I made stupid conversation. I told him I liked the fact that he wore jeans to work. I told him I liked the cover of the book on women's lingerie tacked to his wall. He stopped his pacing and gave me a smirk. I asked him about his tennis. Another smirk. I told him that he should get a science writer to do a piece on Alzheimer's disease.

"What's that?"

Oh, God, I thought, I don't want to explain it. I want to throw up.

"I'll bring you a pamphlet."

"No, no pamphlet. I hate pamphlets. Everybody brings me pamphlets. What is it?"

So I told him everything I knew about it — statistically. I told him it was the worst disease in the world.

"Why do you know so much about it?"

I told him.

"Write me a proposal for that, too."

"What?"

"Write me a proposal for a piece you'll do about your mother, and I'll read the one about the woman who shot her husband, which, by the way, I don't think we'll ever run."

"Oh, no."

"I won't hire a science writer. Come back when you're ready to do it. Now go away."

Everybody but Marty and Howard advised me against it. And from Howard it was the dare I needed. He could write and he was sure I could do it.

Howard took me to buy a new typewriter and then to his house, where we sat up in his study and I typed the two proposals. Again and again.

I handed in both. I looked at my watch. I was sure the one about the woman killing her husband was going to send Marty diving into my office with the eagerness of an editor unearthing a Pulitzer. Eight minutes later he came into my office. There were tears in his eyes.

"Write it," he said, tossing the proposal about my mother on the desk. "Forget the other one."

He had a contract in his hand. He was talking about a fee and expenses and space and a deadline, and I was thinking about my antacids.

During the summer Margaret had begun attending family support groups at New York University Hospital. She was in a group of spouses who lived with victims. She was desperately trying to get me to join a group for children of victims.

She attended the group with spouses because she, too, lived with a victim. It was an interesting concept. My sister, my mother's spouse. My mother, my sister's ward. Margaret, the caretaker. My mother, the bane of my sister's existence. After my mother, me.

I wasn't a great deal of help. I was still clinging to the parental image of my mother. Despite the progress I thought I was making, I was very far from accepting the disease, and my sister and I were growing farther apart by the minute.

"Give up," Margaret said to me. "I can't believe you still think she's going to get better. You're never going to be able to help her if you think that. You're going to continue to ask impossible things of her."

And I did. My mother and I had done some sailing that summer. We went to the club and played tennis and sometimes she would swim. Every Sunday, a morning at the dock and then an afternoon at the pool. Once when she went to the bathroom a man came over and gave me a book about a new type of memory therapy. He said it might help. It was very kind of him. Kinder, much kinder, than the reaction of most other people.

I overheard one person say to another, "Crazy, I hear she's crazy," looking in our direction. I gave the woman a broad smile. I pointed to my mother with a look of question on my face. No? read my expression, not her, and then I pointed to me, with another questioning look. Me, perhaps? And then a smile.

I paraded my mother around and pretended her confusion didn't bother me. Actually, it was driving me crazy. I said that to my mother. I said, "You are driving me crazy," under my breath, teeth clenched, one day when she was tugging on my sleeve, asking me what day it was, and she tugged again and I whipped around on the wide slate of the outdoor patio and she said, "As your father would say, 'That's not a drive, it's a putt,'" smiled, and walked past, while I stood in place in shock. When she was funny, she was a killer.

My mother was a pest. More often than not our day together would be spent with me chasing her around. I would look up and she would be standing with a group of people she recognized, and even from a distance I could read their dismay.

One woman asked me, when I came to retrieve my mother, if I "couldn't control her."

"Under the circumstances," I said, staring at her, "it is unlikely that I can control myself for another instant," and asked my mother to come with me.

I found that people forced me and my sister to say the most devastating things in front of my mother, about her, to explain her behavior. People wanted an explanation, and at first I was unwilling to give it to them. To hell with them, I thought. She's suffering, I'm suffering, Margaret's suffering, let them suffer. Let her grab food off their plates; let her ask them what day it is and how long their husbands have been dead, over and over and over again. I dare them to get up and leave. I dare them to make a sound.

Anyone could have realized that, for the most part, I was simply embarrassed. But if anyone could have realized it, I suppose the first one would have had to be me.

Margaret and I would laugh about it, our image, some of what then could be called my mother's "antics." We had to laugh, because it was so unbearably sad. We were losing separate and different mothers, and my mother was losing herself. My sister was losing a mother, someone she didn't particularly like but who she thought deserved to receive the care our father would have offered. I was losing a mother I idolized and for whom I thought no help would help. Margaret also believed that she should try to spare our mother the embarrassment and indignities of her condition. Margaret felt a moral obligation to care for our mother as best she could while I was still wallowing in panic and despair. I wanted to help, but I didn't know how. I could not see past my grief.

For the most part Allene didn't laugh, although sometimes she made fun of herself.

Following is some dialogue I recorded from that period. It concerns an event that took place at the end of the summer.

ALLENE: What happened to Skip?

MARION: He broke his arm on the boat.

ALLENE: I lost my Nimblet in the hurricane of 1936. Ernie Bilhuber didn't tie it up right. Was I there?

MARION: No.

ALLENE: What happened to Skip?

MARION: Tell me.

ALLENE: He broke his arm on the boat. Is he in the hospital? He's in North Shore. Can we go there? Can we borrow a car?

(We had no car at this time.)

MARION: I made some calls. I am waiting to hear.

ALLENE: The Paulsens have two cars.

MARION: They've gone sailing.

ALLENE: They have two cars.

MARION: But they're not home.

ALLENE: What's wrong with Skip?

MARION: Tell me.

ALLENE: He broke his arm on the boat. Was I there? I had a boat.

MARION: I know.

ALLENE: Was I there?

MARION: No.

ALLENE: I think I was there. I think I started the fire.

MARION: There was no fire and you weren't there.

ALLENE: Should I call the Paulsens?

MARION: No, they've gone sailing.

ALLENE: Tell me once more, what happened to Skip? He broke his arm. How did it happen? Was I there?

MARION: On the boat. He had an accident. We were not there. Jesus, Ma, let's change the subject.

ALLENE: What's new?

MARION: I've been working.

ALLENE: What do you do?

MARION: I'm a news assistant in the Travel section at the *Times.*

ALLENE: What is that?

MARION: I do charts and graphs and do some work with pictures.

ALLENE: What's wrong with Skip?

(I look at the floor.)

ALLENE: He broke his arm on the boat. Was I there?

MARION: You're not trying. You have to try to remember. You can remember. You're not trying.

ALLENE: I am. I'm very trying.

(She smiles and lights a cigarette.)

The long hall of the Milhauser Clinic at New York University Medical Center is busy. Some people shuffle. Some sit, staring at the walls. Quiet conversation at the water fountain consists of questions.

"Is he agitated?"

"Does she sleep through the night?"

"Does he speak?"

Family members compare patients, making mental notes, one instant elated and the next devastated by the differences. One may walk but not speak. Another is conversational but violent. Another just paces, up and down the hall, back and forth, shaking his head. The first time I sat there in that long hall, I didn't know, as I looked from face to face, if I was looking at a victim of the disease or a family member, a victim of being related to a victim. A victim's victim.

In the same hall is a depression program. Many times, I have thought of jumping into one of their groups, instead. I was very depressed. I have since learned just how depressed. A recent study of family members of those with this disease revealed that 50 percent suffer from what is known as primary depression. The behavioral concomitants were painfully familiar to me at this time, but I didn't know there was a name for the condition.

When I told Margaret that I was going to write the piece about Allene, she said that I was "opening Pandora's box." She suggested that if I really wanted to do it, I should join a support group. I joined one run by Gert Steinberg and Emma Shulman, and within the first two hours I decided to put my heart in their hands. Emma is the size of a pint of good cold milk, and Gert has the biggest heart in the world. But the descriptions are interchangeable; they are both small and fierce and devoted.

There was a long table of ten. I sat and listened to one woman say that her mother had gone that week into a nursing home. Her eyes were spilling tears, and she looked tired. Roberta's mother is fifty-seven and doesn't speak; she shrieks, especially when anyone tries to put her in the shower. Jewel's husband couldn't figure out his keys. I was home. This was the stuff that I needed to hear. It was a banquet of guilt and remorse and sadness, and for the first time in three years I wasn't alone.

"Why are you here?" Emma asked about an hour into the meeting, after I had heard some other descriptions.

I became hot and, I knew, red from the neck up. I mumbled something. I did not say that I was writing about it. I felt ashamed. All of a sudden, I didn't feel like such an expert. Not if it had taken me this long to realize I needed help.

My sister and I had gotten to the point of thinking that somehow we deserved our mother's disease. It was a drudgery we had come to accept. And in accepting it, we were accepting the solitary confinement of shame. We were ashamed of her — her actions, her speech, her manners — and we were ashamed of ourselves for not having a healthy mother. Cancer was all right, almost, or heart disease, but a mental disorder, now that was something to be ashamed of.

Margaret and I became close friends with Dr. Barry Reisberg, the clinical psychiatrist who was caring for our mother. Margaret had been taking Allene to see him on a regular basis since the original diagnosis.

I do not know if it is Barry's nature to be gentle and patient with every person he sees, but to us he was a kind and observant professional and a good and honest friend. He understood completely — unlike so many other doctors I have met — that this disease takes more than one victim;

that it takes the family as well and creates a new and wholly unstable environment around all concerned. We developed an attachment to him that transcended any I have ever expected of a doctor-patient relationship. Slowly and considerately he had convinced us of the value of his research into the clinical aspects of this disease, so when he asked us to bring our mother to be observed by some of his students, we readily agreed.

I am very nervous. My mother is pacing, asking where she is, why she is here, and what day it is. My sister keeps telling me that this is an important project, that at least Dr. Reisberg's students will benefit. I guess I look as if I don't believe it.

We are asked into a small room filled with young students. One student is asking another, "Advisers, we're supposed to have advisers? Do I have one? Oh, God, I didn't know I needed an adviser."

I wish I were back in college. I wish I were back in college and my father was alive and my sister was living in New York and, oh well . . .

"Sure you have one. He may not see you, he may not know you from Adam, but you got one, useless as they are."

Over the conversation I hear, "Why are we here? What kinds of questions is he going to ask me?"

"Just questions, Mommy," says Margaret.

"Like what day is it?" asks my mother, leaning into my sister's face.

"Yes, that's right."

"What day is it?" My mother is cramming for her exam. She is very, very nervous. Her eyes search me out in the room. I am sitting at the other end of a long table. I want to observe. I take notes. Whenever I am nervous, I scribble in a notebook. These days I go through a lot of notebooks.

Dr. Reisberg introduces Mrs. Roach.

My mother smiles.

"The purpose of this gathering is to meet Mrs. Roach, who is a patient of mine with a memory problem," says Dr. Reisberg. He has given out questionnaires to the students to evaluate her answers and to assess the level of her problem.

He turns to her. "Do you know where you are?"

"Yes."

"Where are you?"

"The medical center."

"How do you feel?"

"A little nervous. I am afraid I am going to embarrass myself because of my memory loss."

I want to cry.

"How do you feel about your memory loss?"

"I haven't gotten used to the idea. It is restructuring my life. I can't drive a car."

"Since when?"

"About a year."

"Is this true?" Dr. Reisberg asks, looking at Margaret.

"No, it's been only three months," says Margaret, looking right at him.

Boy, she's better at this than I am, I think, as she continues and says, "She stopped driving about three months ago. We had to take away the keys. She got lost on the expressway for four and a half hours."

It's true, but I wasn't told until several days later. She was on her way to Bay Shore. Her friend Elise was waiting at the exit ramp. Margaret had the police looking for her all afternoon. Margaret had taken to noting the mileage before she left and when she returned, a new habit formed almost without notice. Another new device for gauging the disease. I knew about that, because I did it when I was there. Spies together. On that day, Allene must have been driving the whole time, although Margaret didn't know where. After Margaret told me about the incident, we took away the keys and sold the car. It was a horrible experience. Allene was angry and resentful and she tried to steal keys to a borrowed car from my purse, but I caught her on her way out the door. When I asked her where she was going, she stopped at the front door, clutched her purse to her heart, and just said, "Away."

They are still talking. I have been staring out the window.

"Mrs. Roach, when did your memory problem start?"

"About a year ago," my mother replies. She looks at Dr. Reisberg and asks in a begging, imploring voice that makes me shiver, "What is wrong with me?"

"You tell me," he says. He doesn't miss a beat, thank God. I am crying.

"What did I have, a stroke?" my mother asks, again in an imploring tone.

"Well, how has it affected you?" he asks.

"I can't drive my car. I can't go anywhere by myself. I am kind of resentful. I had to give up driving about a year ago."

"When did all this happen, this memory problem? When did it start?" Dr. Reisberg asks.

"About a year ago. It seemed to happen suddenly, to occur immediately. Sometimes my short-term memory is nonexistent."

"Have you ever had any medical problems?"

"No."

"Is this true?" Again he turns to Margaret.

"Three years ago she suffered from terrible depression. She went through menopause and had a tough time after being diagnosed as having a precancerous condition. She had a hysterectomy. She has a history of drinking. She has a slight heart condition, a mitral valve prolapse."

Allene stares at Margaret. She just stares at her, in what looks like shock. I am trying to read her look. It is blank, but it is angry.

"Where are you?" Dr. Reisberg asks my mother.

"I," my mother says defiantly, staring at Margaret, "am in Manhattan at the New York University Medical Center," and then nods, like punctuation.

Go for it, Ma.

"Do you know the date?"

Pause. Stares into space. Quietly, "No."

"The year?"

"Nineteen eighty-two."

Right, go on, now tell me you're faking the whole thing and let's leave and we'll forget all about this.

"The month?"

"Summer. August, the middle of the month."

She goes on to tell him her address, complete with zip code, her phone number with area code, and that she came to the city in a small red car.

She doesn't know what she did this morning. Margaret says she went swimming.

My mother says she doesn't read the news. She says she cannot remember the word before the one she has just read, so she doesn't get very far, but she used to read and worked for a newspaper and she married the slowest writer in the press box at the racetrack. And then she smiles.

She is asked to subtract four from forty and eventually gets down to sixteen and then says she can't go any further.

"I see. That's fine, though," says Dr. Reisberg. "Now what number did you start with?"

"What? I don't remember."

"Do you cry?"

"No."

She looks up at the student who asked the question. The students have been asked to interview her. "But you know what?" she says, looking right at him, after a hesitation. "This whole thing makes me think about the past a lot, how good things used to be, and I think I'm depressed."

There is a lull.

A young man says to her, "Mrs. Roach, don't look down, but tell me what those initials on your shirt mean?"

"G.B. you mean?" she asks. She hasn't looked down. "Geoffrey Beene." She flashes a winning smile.

Grace under pressure. She could rewrite the book.

Class dismissed. We go out into the hall, my sister, our mother, and I. We are told to wait a few minutes. My sister and I are shaking our heads.

"Did I pass?" my mother asks, snapping her gum like a coed and then making a turn for the bathroom. Is she kidding? Is she being serious? Sarcastic? Margaret and I stand there and look after my mother on her way into the bathroom.

"I can't believe it," I say. "I don't get it."

At home she turns on the gas jets, feeds the three surviving cats seven times a day, wakes my sister up four, five times a night to ask what day it is, and here she knows the name of some damn designer. I fear the students must think we are awful, must think there is nothing wrong with her that new — different — daughters wouldn't cure. Of course, I have forgotten that she answered every question about the past by saying "about a year ago" and that she didn't remember the name of anyone who was at her wedding.

My mother is still in the bathroom. My sister and I are talking. "They must think we are real shrews," Margaret says. "God, I feel like a shit."

"Me too."

My mother comes bursting out of the bathroom. Her purse is open and things are spilling out onto the floor. Half of her head has been combed. The other half is a tangled mess.

"What day is it?" she asks, clutching me, sinking her nails into my forearm.

Chapter 10

"ARE YOU really getting married?" I shout into the phone. It was just a few weeks after the appointment with Dr. Reisberg and his students, on a Sunday.

A good friend from college is on the other end of the phone.

"God, really? You and Andrew? I can't believe it. I mean, I can, of course, but I can't. You know. Oh, God."

My mother is hovering over me, breathing the smoke from her fifth cigarette of the morning into the stiff collar of my shirt.

"I married your father because he was the slowest writer in the press box," my mother says to no one.

I look at her with, I am sure, disbelief. I mean, I'm on the phone and she's ignoring that. "Ma, I'm on the phone."

"He used to sit with his fingers in his hair and gasp and stare at the typewriter. I married him because he was the slowest writer in the press box."

"I know, Ma."

Ella Fitzgerald is wafting through the speakers in the kitchen. The record clicks to a finish.

"Ma, why don't you go change the record, okay?"

Back to the phone. My mother drifts from the room.

"Jane, this is great. When's the wedding?"

I cannot hear the answer. The record is blaring. My mother has started the record again, on the same side, but turned the volume way up.

"Wait a minute, Jane."

I dash out to the sun porch, turn down the volume, and bring my mother to the kitchen with me.

Back to the phone, again with my mother hovering over me, staring at nothing.

"Okay, Jane, so when's the wedding?"

"I married your father because he was the slowest writer in the press box."

"Hold on a sec, Jane. Ma, please, I'll be right off."

She stares blankly at my forehead.

"Nothing, Jane, no, my mother was just telling me something. Jane, that's great, really."

At Jane's backyard wedding, several months later, there were fifty people. I saw a lot of college friends. Two of them had relatives who were Alzheimer's victims. Casual conversation, this and that, brought out that three of us knew more about this disease than we wanted to know. Three in fifty.

My father was a journalist. My mother had been one; my sister too. I thought that with a Chesterfield coat from Brooks Brothers and a typewriter, you could re-create anybody's life for a reader.

At the beginning of September I began interviewing doctors for my magazine assignment. Peter Davies was the first. Dr. Davies is a neuropathologist at the Albert Einstein College of Medicine. He studies brain tissue. We looked at test tubes and we chain-smoked cigarettes. I had started smoking again after more than a year.

I liked Dr. Davies very much. I didn't expect to. The word "pathology" has always conjured up for me images of a dungeon, of Frankenstein. And a neuropathologist, I thought, was the worst of the bunch; he takes brains. I was sure he would want to delight me with parts of a real brain and that he would have one sealed in a jar on his desk, if he wasn't sitting smugly in front of a bookcase full of them.

He did nothing of the sort. He was dedicated to and in love with his work and very able to explain it to anyone who was interested. We spent about three hours together. He told me about writing grant proposals, and he worked on the blackboard, drawing the neurons to look as they should, like trees, and next to that picture, drawing them with their branches all tangled: the healthy brain, the diseased brain.

I started thinking of my mother's brain filled with tangles and neuritic plaques. It was hard for me to imagine, until I remembered what Todd had told me about the brain, about how it is all electric circuits, and that sometimes they just burn out. I started thinking that my mother had some sort of short circuit and that she needed rewiring.

I tried, obviously, to humanize all the notions, to simplify the terminology to myself, to clear away that misunderstanding — that a disease happens only to other people, in other people's poorly structured limbs and organs.

I felt like a spy. In some interviews I told the doctors about my mother. In others, I kept it to myself. I felt that they might tell something to a professional writer that they wouldn't tell a child of a victim.

I had interviewed Lewis Thomas, the science writer and chancelor of Memorial Sloan-Kettering. He said that this was the "disease of the century, because of all the health problems in the twentieth century, this one is the worst."

After interviewing Dr. Davies, I interviewed Robert Katzman at Einstein. Then I went to New York University Medical Center and interviewed Dr. Reisberg, Dr. Mony de Leon, and Dr. Ravi Anand. I finished my research by the end of October.

Whenever I asked about the cause, I tried to look nonchalant, because by this point, every time I lost my keys or forgot someone's first name, I thought that the disease was in the blood. I would ask the question and hope for something definite, something conclusive. I didn't get it.

ANAND: My gut reaction is that it's not genetic; more metabolic, some degree of immune incompetency.

REISBERG: I have no gut feeling, but I can describe what happens. The genetic aspects have been overemphasized, to the consternation of the families. I'm looking for blood tests, immunological changes in the blood. Toxic causes are not convincing. I am more concerned with treatment.

THOMAS: If I had to bet — and I wouldn't bet real money — I'd bet on it being a slow virus.

DAVIES: If it's a gene, all you have to do is delay its expression, delay it twenty years. If it's a virus, it's a bloody strange beast.

I became very gun-shy. I became afraid of subways and of my apartment. I was jittery. I developed a terrible fear of the phone and would disconnect it from the wall when I was home. I had surrounded myself with the subject, visiting my mother on Sundays and writing about it every day, going to my meetings on Wednesday nights, and working to expand the Alzheimer's Disease and Related Disorders Association with Margaret.

After my regular job at the *Times* during the day, I would stay and sit with Marianne at nearby desks and write until three in the morning. She always worked late, and we spent six months together, at night, eating junk, ripping through packs of cigarettes, and giving each other complete support.

Mary had moved back to Paris right at the time I took the assignment. Her absence stunned me. We went out to dinner at the Odeon with a pack of friends on her last night, and then she was gone. I missed her desperately.

Marianne was fiercely loyal about families. There were no secrets in her home. The first time I went to dinner there, it took an hour or so for me to become adjusted to the strong personalities and the constant and loud conversation at the dinner table; everybody yelled, not in anger, but to make sure they got their opinions heard. They yelled in Greek. So I just ate and ate. When they finally lapsed into English, I joined right in. Marianne's mother was convinced that Marianne and I were "holding out" against marriage. Every time we mentioned a man's name — a co-worker, a friend — she'd scream, "Marry him." I went with Nicky there for dinner once, and Mrs. Costantinou leaped, orally, from one to the other of us, trying to talk him into it, me, Marianne.

My loyal sweet friend Marianne had a terribly hard time dealing with my mother's illness. She told me that she could always listen but that she didn't think she ever wanted to go with me to visit. I respected that totally. There was no reason for her to see my mother. She never put me off in my despair, and her honesty was more important to me than her witnessing something that she could not have completely understood.

For the six months it took me to write the piece, Marianne and I sat back to back, typing and groaning, smoking and pounding our fists. She wrote story after story as I plodded along with the one. In that time we never went to the movies or to dinner or saw each other on weekends. We just worked.

Another person who listened and watched was Annie. Annie started at the *Times* a year after I did. After my family support meetings I would take a cab to her perfect little apartment next to St. Patrick's and she would feed me beers. Annie doesn't really drink, but she always had two six-packs in her tiny fridge for her pal. I would just show up on a Wednesday evening or on a Saturday afternoon, and she'd be ready. One Saturday I showed up twice, the second time without warning. She had already replenished her supply. Annie had a mother with the most predictable habit of calling every night at eleven. I was terribly jealous of those calls, and yet very happy to overhear a wonderful mother-daughter relationship.

Mary had been the friend with whom I went dancing or to galleries or parties, and when she left I didn't think of replacing her. I didn't go out with girls at all. Annie and Marianne listened and wept.

It was with Tracy that I had my most tempestuous relationship. One night, early into my writing the magazine piece, Tracy called and said she was coming over. I was working at home for once. She said she didn't care if she was disturbing me; she had to see me.

She marched in the door and pointed her finger at me. She said that she thought I was doing the right thing, but that I was doing it all wrong. She was making an assumption that infuriated me. I fought with her, and then she began to ask questions. Without reading any of the article, she had made a perfect assessment of my vision of it. I was probably being too particular, she said, and not thinking of the larger picture. Personal was fine, detail is wonderful. But, she maintained, it is easy to walk away from a disease, from any heartbreak, if you find a detail in the reading or the telling that allows you to disqualify yourself, to believe it can never happen to you.

She was right. I began to realize that people are fascinated by "madness." Everyone wants to know what it looks like, how it feels, and how it starts. It's more complicated than simple rubber-necking. Some people seem to believe that if they have every detail, they can prevent themselves from ever worrying about it. Other people, however, have a resigned attitude toward it, and they want to know the symptoms so that they'll know it when they see it coming.

Very soon after my father died I had flown out to Michigan to see a friend from college. I was a wreck. As we lay on the floor in his living room, talking the way the closest of friends do, he asked me what it "looked like" when my father was in a coma. I will never forget what it looked like, how his body convulsed, how he gasped for air through his puckered, rounded mouth. My friend pushed me for every detail. I hadn't thought about it until Tracy and I explored this notion. It was a magical help, because until then I was writing to wipe out my grief and my guilt, and at her insistence I saw that I had to write with other people in mind.

By November the writing was going well. The article was almost finished. I took an evening off from writing to go to Douglaston to vote. We vote in the auditorium of the grammar school my mother attended. My mother's card was in front of mine in that dark, thick, heavy, long-leaf book of yellow cards. The cards make the pages soft waves of the Christian names of people you know as Neal but who are really Cornelius when you look close. I saw the deterioration of my signature over the years, and I thought of my father.

I looked again, saw my mother's name, and felt no hope. I remembered how she used to go to vote at the grammar school Margaret and I attended. She would leave us in the car, and when she came out she always had a cake or cookies. There was a bake sale at the same time as the voting.

My mother had loved to vote. She said it was a very important thing to do. When we were kids, she said if Nixon won over Kennedy, she was going to pack us up and leave the country. She said it while we were dissolving hunks of angel food cake in our mouths in the car after she had voted.

As I stood looking at the long yellow pages and my mother's signature, I thought of going home and getting her and taking her into the voting booth with me. But I knew that it would never work for either one of us. She was too agitated. I took a train back to the city twenty minutes after I arrived.

On the train to Manhattan I thought about the woman who, just as I was leaving, came in for her shift of supervising the polls. She looked like an older version of her daughter, who is six years older than I. I realized that they had always had the same taste for large earrings, and I wondered how much I looked like my mother.

On Thanksgiving my mother and I were invited to the home of Tom and Lette. There were twenty-four people in a room that has seen three generations of a family. Around the table were dishes of cranberry ice from the recipe of Marion Rollins Zillmann, for whom I am named.

My mother had talked about the ice from the beginning of November. She thought she had made the one we brought, but it was Margaret, who, late the night before, had been there to take over when it proved an impossible task. My mother couldn't boil the water to make the cranberries soft. She didn't know how to boil water, but there were cranberries everywhere.

Her conversation for three weeks before the dinner was of cranberry ice and nonalcoholic wine. The night before, she said nothing but "Ah, ah, cranberry ice, nonalcoholic wine, and Scotch." These were the things she was to bring to the dinner. There was no sentence, no phrase other than that, over and over.

It was a cheerful, glorious dinner. It was loud, and Lette seated me far enough away from my mother so that she herself fielded most of Mother's questions, and we all laughed and ate.

Later, my mother said she had a nice time. She didn't remember that she wouldn't sit still — would barely sit down for more than a moment — until her cranberry ice was on the table. Then she became even more agitated. She kept telling people that theirs was melting. She said it to everyone, again and again. Then she asked the woman next to her why she wasn't eating hers, and the woman dutifully ate hers in several scoops. My mother turned to her and said, "Didn't you like it?" The woman nodded yes, and my mother asked, "Then why didn't you eat it?"

She didn't remember that she continued to get upset and that we left early. We were exhausted. We went to her home and put on our matching flannel down-to-the-floor nightgowns and went to bed at eight.

Right before Christmas, Margaret went to Jamaica for a week with a friend of ours from high school. I was glad. Ever since Gregory had moved out nine months earlier, she had seemed lonely. I kept expecting him to reappear, but he didn't.

While Margaret was away I stayed with my mother. One night, while we were having dinner at the club at our table for two, which hugs a huge mirror, I asked her about her marriage.

"I married your father because he was the slowest writer in the press box."

"I know, Ma, but really, I mean, tell me about marriage." I thought it was something she might want to discuss, something she would be able to, because it was in the past.

Instead, she quickly said the names of two ex-boyfriends of Margaret's, one of whom none of us had heard from in six years. On any one subject her words came out like boxcars hurtling down an incline, out of control.

I was getting nowhere, but I was desperate, so I pursued the subject. It became a matter of locked knowledge: I wanted to know what makes a relationship work. I thought she had the secret locked up in there somewhere, and I was going to find it. I needed it. I brought up the topic again. Again, the same response, about the press box.

I started to cry. I reached across and held her forearm. "Ma, please, there's no one else for me to ask. Please, Mom, I'm so unhappy about the relationships I've had, and I don't know what I do wrong."

The conversation had slipped dangerously from something I thought she would enjoy talking about to some huge, gaping need of mine.

"I married your father because he was the slowest writer in the press box," she said, looking at her salad.

In December my mother began getting injections of a new drug that was being tested by Dr. Reisberg. Testing done at the clinic at New York University Medical Center had resulted in some encouraging results. The clinic, which Dr. Reisberg headed, did diagnoses, referrals, maintenance, and drug-testing as well as running the family support groups. Independently Barry saw those patients who were ineligible for the clinic program.

The programs were funded mostly by the drug companies, which, understandably, maintained certain requirements for admission. Patients could be excluded if they had heart conditions or a history of alcoholism, for example. The purpose was not only to protect the patients but also to ensure that no other complicating illness confused the results of the research.

My mother had been excluded because of her drinking. Margaret had taken her for the evaluation. If I had taken her, I am sure that I never would have mentioned it. To Margaret, it seemed another illness.

Dr. Reisberg was administering the injections at his private office. He gave the first one in the middle of the month. Following the shot and a waiting period of forty minutes, Mom was given questions to answer. She was as confused and agitated as she had been without the drug, and she failed — as she had before the injection — her "test," for which we had crammed. I had told her what day it was and what time it was. She was nervous and fidgety but seemed totally unaware of day-to-day matters.

She was asked to write a sentence. She wrote, "Merry Christmas." I was surprised and pleased. Dr. Reisberg asked her to write something longer. She wrote, "I have a memory problem." I felt tears fill my eyes.

I was told to be aware of any change in her behavior after we left. She and I went for a little lunch and then for the drive home. It was about two hours after the injection. She was just as repetitive, but violently and relentlessly more agitated than I had ever seen her. In the snow, on the FDR Drive, she tried to wrest the steering wheel from me because I wouldn't pay enough attention to her. I was alone with her, trying to drive in a swirl of snow, and she wanted me to look at her when I answered her questions.

When I spoke with Dr. Reisberg the following day, he was very concerned. The next week at my Wednesday night Alzheimer's support group meeting, Gert said that "as soon as you lose communication, the grief begins."

She was right. It was beginning to sink in. My mother and I were losing touch. I had blocked out what had happened that day, right before the incident on the FDR Drive. But now, with her words about communication, it made sense, and it came back like a wrecked car the next day in the driveway.

When we left Dr. Reisberg's, on our way to lunch, we had walked along the East River in the snow. We passed a girl who might have been nine — a redhead, like me — swaying under the weight of wrapped packages. When I was a child, my mother would point out adult redheads and tell me whether or not she hoped I would grow up to look like them. As I got older, she would point out children and tell me whether I had looked like them. It was a routine.

She passed the package-laden girl without a word. I tried to begin our routine, saying, "Another redhead." My mother looked straight ahead.

The communication was gone. I realized it then, and I had blocked it. As fast as it had gotten in, I pushed it out. Now I knew that my mother and I would never again have that on-the-bed, stomach-down, real-truth time together. It was during one of those times that I had decided my favorite color was green, because she said it was hers.

My favorite color is still green.

Christmas almost passed like a blur. It was very sad. My mother tore through packages and grabbed for more. Sometimes she had trouble opening the boxes and would grip them at the edges, turning them slowly in her hands. She would stare at them. It was clear that she did not know what to do with them, what they were. Then that moment would pass and she would tear at them with a vengeance.

The article on my mother was printed in the *New York Times* Sunday magazine on January 16, 1983. It began with the incident about the cats. I have never been able to get out of my head the image of her holding them. I have never seen anything, ever since, that shocked me more. The first slash is the worst. The piece went on to describe her changes and give details about the research being conducted on Alzheimer's disease. The magazine is always ready on the Wednesday night before the Sunday it hits the stands. I went to my group meeting that Wednesday and gave the other members a copy and then went home and held the magazine in my hands almost until I fell asleep.

On Sunday I was with my mother. We had an appointment with Dr. Reisberg for another injection; he sees patients seven days a week. I had driven out, picked her up, driven back into the city, then out again.

The appointment had not gone well. Again, she was very agitated following the injection. It was frustrating to be with Dr. Reisberg and not be able to discuss the magazine piece. I wanted to know whether he thought the medical aspects of it were correct. I hadn't told my mother about it. She couldn't read it. She couldn't read.

She was very concerned about the traffic on the way back, how she had done on her test at the doctor's, about the traffic, the test, whose car it was, over and over. I was happy to get her home and return to the city. It was a very special day for me. I thought it would be the beginning of the end of my grief.

It wasn't. She was still sick, and I felt very alone. The next day I started getting calls from people and the day after some offers to turn the article into a book. I was very confused. I was also stunned by the attention. I had thought that we were so very alone with our problem.

I had always imagined that on the day — whenever it was — that I had my first success, however I judged it, I would have someone, a parent most specifically, there to coo, as my Dad had when I first started at the *Times*. My mother didn't know anything about it, my father was dead, and my sister was undecided about her feelings. She wanted to wait for the reaction. I felt like a brat, wanting more attention, and then in an instant I just wanted some celebration. I used to get that from my mother.

Several friends of my mother were very critical about my being so personal in public. My sister received some vicious hang-up calls. I was amazed.

Addie Millington, a friend of my mother's, called. I remembered her from my youth, but I hadn't seen her in twenty years. She and my mother had kept in touch and had lunched in the city over the years. They had originally met at the racetrack when my parents were first married. Addie told me that she had read the piece and that it explained a great deal. My mother had broken a few dates with her in the last year and, Addie told me, Allene was very confused when they saw each other last, maybe a year before this call. She wanted to have lunch with me.

Addie looked very much the way I remembered her. She was now a successful photographer, living in New Jersey and working in New York. She was very interested in my mother's condition, but she was more interested in the condition of Margaret and me. She was guarded, a little, on the subject of my mother.

I said, I remember quite well, that "it is interesting, intellectually, as a daughter, to discover so much about my mother. There are so many things I would never know about if it weren't for this. But I do, and that's that. You know what I mean?"

She did. She knew that Janet Kaplan, for instance, was a cover. She knew that Janet Kaplan had been created when I was eight. Not even I was sure just what age I was when it started. I knew that "she" had been around for a long time, but it didn't hit so hard as when I thought of myself as eight and I thought of my mother having a life outside our home, a life that may have included a romance.

Addie and I began seeing each other for lunch on something of a schedule. She also began visiting my mother regularly. At our third lunch I was very uncomfortable. I kept trying to steer the conversation away from the mother-daughter relationship, yet, with the same determination, I wanted it there. I had conditioned myself to accept that there was no longer a mother for me, that there were to be no chats, no secrets about love or bras, questions about morality or fashion.

And yet I pined for it. I heard this voice speaking — mine — about the details of life, about my love life, and at the same time I felt a desire to cut it off, to hold back. This was not my mother sitting across from me at lunch at Harvey's

— one of my favorite saloons — over the best fried oysters in New York. This was a woman with a life of her own who would be getting on a train tonight, back to New Jersey, back to her family, and I would have told my secrets to someone who wouldn't fully understand.

Addie wanted to know what I planned to write next. She took my career seriously. I was having trouble with the decision. I didn't know quite what I wanted to write, but she assumed that I intended to keep writing, just as my mother would have done had she been there. There was no question to her. I had a career. To me, there was every question about everything. I hinted about sex, about my wondering what it's all about, about if that's all there is in a relationship, and if you're sure you are unhappy in the relationship, whether you should stay anyway. She jumped right in about things being so good and healthy these days and people having the right attitude and how you can get good sex elsewhere. We talked on and on, and when I went home I felt terribly abandoned and alone.

I have always felt that if you manage to get something up from the heart, through the brain, and out the mouth, you'd better be prepared to relive it — smell it, feel it, see it again. If you don't want to revive it, I figure, don't talk about it.

Good old Holden Caulfield, with his "never tell anybody anything or you'll start missing everybody."

You bet.

I miss my mother. I miss her in a dangerous way. I want her. I want my father, dammit. I want to go for a stroll with both of them and talk.

They were on a stroll — my father and mother — when she explained to him about kissing. Girls, after one age and before another, she explained, don't like to be kissed. Not (and this was the painful part) by their fathers.

When Margaret and I were small, my father had a favorite

game. It was our favorite game, too. He was the Kissing Bandit. He would tie his large white handkerchief, which smelled of starch, around his head, right on the tip of his nose and over his mouth. He was the only bandit I ever saw who wore Brooks Brothers trousers while he prowled.

My sister and I would be lying next to each other in our small beds, our knees up, whispering about some adventure, about Eloise or Pippi Longstocking, and we would hear the stairs creak.

Another small creak.

One of us would dive under the covers. One might make it into the closet, amid the rubber boots and pinafores, but the creaking would continue. And then the growling warning from the Kissing Bandit that he was coming for his due.

There was no hiding. The screaming always gave away the best-hidden daughter, and he would find us and scoop us out of our places and kiss us through the handkerchief, and in those eyes over the cloth there was such a look of complete and gentle delighted love that it was all right.

Until a certain age. Margaret held on as long as she could. I think she did it for me. At about eight years of age, she didn't particularly like being kissed — and my father kissed, God forbid, in public — but she put up with it, as with Santa and the Easter Bunny, for me. When I gave in to its being icky, however, it stopped.

My mother took my father for a walk around the neighborhood, and after that there was kissing only when he couldn't stop himself. Sometimes it was clear that a kiss was on the way, and then he would stop — hesitate — with a look of disappointment and pat us on the head.

My mother had interceded. And that was that.

Chapter 11

WHEN I SAT DOWN in August 1982 to write the magazine article, I had taken a first step in the proper direction. I was coming around. Or at least I was coming to terms with the disease, with the end of my relationship with my mother as I had known it, with the end of those real-truth times together as the mother and daughter I so desperately wanted us to be. I had described her as she had been and I had described her as she was. I discussed her future in terms of possible loss of speech, incontinence, and death.

When the piece was publishd the following January, I thought I was done with it. I had done my wash in public, and I felt a momentary elation. But the depression that followed was stunning. My mother wasn't any better.

It seemed simple enough, but apparently I hadn't learned a great deal about grief. I hadn't even come to terms with the fact that I was grieving. My mother was still sick and I was still floundering.

I was appallingly listless at work. I was resentful of the smallest duty. And it got tougher every day. The woman with whom I worked lived with her elderly mother. Shortly before, her mother had fallen and broken her hip. She had eye problems, but a marvelous spirit. Ursula lived with her and cared for her, and I was feeling guilty as hell every day for not living with my mother — only visiting on Sundays — and then for having written about it. I felt like a fake. I had received more than five hundred letters and four hundred phone calls following the magazine piece. I have those letters. Any one picked at random relates a similar life, locked in the environment of this relentless disease. Each has phrases like "a holocaust of the mind," a disease of the spirit as well as the brain." Some begin with accounts of incontinence, of wandering, of personal failures, and personal and devastating grief.

I treasure this one.

Dear Miss Roach,

There are a lot of things in this world that piss me off. What's really bothering me today is that I don't understand why I'm sitting in my room in the barracks and I want to cry. You see, as a 25-year-old noncommissioned officer in the U.S. Army (I'm stationed at West Point, where I work in the TV studio), I'm not supposed to get emotional very easily. After all I've actually run towards live machine gun fire, been gassed, and have plastic explosive go off close enough to pick me up off the ground and throw me back down. These things I find easy.

What I find difficult is the way I feel after reading your article in the Sunday *Times Magazine*. The tough part is that I know what's really got me upset. It's not the article itself, or even that I want to cry. I'm mad because I'm not crying when I want to, when I feel like it.

So please don't apologize to your readers and yourself for crying while you and your sister watch your mother die. I fought back the tears when, at the age of seventeen, I graduated from high school just in time to learn that my father was going to die of ALS, or Lou Gehrig's disease . . . He had been getting progressively weaker for several years, but I tried to ignore it; but now he was in a wheelchair and I was the only one to push it. (My sister was away in college, my brother's grown and moved away.) Later, I'd have to wash him, feed him, clean up his vomit, and help him go to the toilet. After two years of this I sat in a hospital room for three days and held his hand as I watched him die. I was mad then too, and I fought the tears as hard as I could. When I get all of this out of my system and write it down, do you know what happens? I start to cry. So I'll close now and take satisfaction in my own ability to feel — something I'll never be ashamed of. Good luck. You're a very brave young woman.

I didn't feel very brave.

The phone calls were back to back. What can I do? Where can I go?

God, I wanted to know the same thing. And then came this one. "Hello, I am seventy-six years old and I live alone in the Bronx. My husband died twelve years ago. I maintain my own apartment and I have nothing wrong with my mind, nothing wrong with my ability to get around. I am self-sufficient."

"Hello." It was the first time she took even a little break so that I could get a word in.

"I want to talk to you."

"Okay."

"I read your article."

"Yes."

"I learned a lot."

"Thank you."

"But there is something I didn't learn. My daughter is fifty-four. Like your mother. Fifty-four. My daughter is in a nursing home. My daughter isn't self-sufficient. My daughter has something wrong with her brain. My daughter is senile. Do you know what it's like to put your daughter in a nursing home? Can you tell me how to feel about that?"

No, I couldn't.

We are born knowing that we will outlive our parents. Her problem was a ghoulish, unforgivable inversion.

After the article was reprinted in several newspapers, letters started coming in again. People thanked me for letting them cry. A professor of psychiatry wrote to say that he was copying the article and making it required reading for his courses. In Canada, Florida, and Milwaukee, people opened the door a crack to their experiences with a disability that is too embarrassing to have anyone see. Almost every other letter began with "This is the first time I have told anyone this, but," and then there would be an account of soiled clothes, a disappearance in the rain, a mother at the wedding not knowing her daughter, the bride.

Of the people who phoned, many asked to come and talk with me. I refused all of them. I didn't think of myself as educated enough to give lengthy advice, and I didn't want to impose on a stranger to give the advice that was offered. Then I got one call from a man who sounded so desperate but so sane that I gave in.

We met for lunch. He was tall and middle-aged and seemed calm but unhappy. We sat down at a place a block from the *Times*.

He said, "You know, it all karma," and proceeded to try to get me to join an expensive mystic group whose belief was based on the premise that all disease is wished for — by the victim.

My friend Francis Martin called me from Washington. He is not afraid to wield the icepick when necessary. He told me I sounded like a wreck. It was eleven at night, and I was home answering letters, the same thing I had been doing nearly every night for three weeks. I was crying.

Some of the letters were beautiful. I got a packet from the fifth grade of a school in Queens — one from each student — that took me five months to answer, because every time

I sat down and started a reply, I stopped, unable to deal with the writers' delicate honesty.

I read some to Francis.

"Are you sure you should answer them?" he asked.

I was sure.

"I think," he suggested, "that you are suffering from a little self-importance. I think you need a sense of humor." I had lost my sense of humor. He was right.

"Let me tell you a little story," he said. "My grandmother was senile. Probably she had Alzheimer's disease. Her husband, who loved her very, very much, took care of her. He kept their wedding picture next to the bed, always within arm's reach, on his side. Every night when he came out of the bathroom after washing up for bed, his wife of more than fifty years would sit up like a whip and ask, 'Who are you?' and demand that he leave her bedroom, and every night he would go to the wedding photo and point to the bride and say, 'Who's that?' and she would smile and say, 'Me,' and then he would point to the groom and say, 'Who's that?' and she would smile and say, 'That's you.' And then she would give him a look as if to tell him to stop all this nonsense and say, 'Now go to sleep.'

"He had a sense of humor, Marion, or else it never would have worked."

My sister sent me a Valentine's card that had a weird-looking person on the front. It read, "Before We Become Valentines, You Should Know There's Insanity in My Family . . ." and inside said, "I'm Crazy About You."

My sister still had her sense of humor.

Our constant help continued. Sharon, the young woman we sponsored from Grenada, worked as a housekeeper for Margaret as well as a companion for my mother. Eva still came and stayed with my mother, but at seventy-six years of age she no longer did housework. Eva was beautifully protective of my mother. Unfortunately, she was jealous of any attention my mother paid to Sharon, and she criticized Sharon continually. Sometimes the feud was a nice distraction. If I went to sit down, Eva would shriek, "Don't sit there; Sharon sat there!" And she would push me aside and beat the cushion, exorcising the spirit. It was very interesting to me. Eva had been around for years, but I did not get to know her at all until this time. I suppose until then I thought nothing at all of her devotion. She was spirited and determined and truly loved my mother. We would sit and talk and I found out all about her life. I was amused by the jealousy between the two women. I was glad that my mother could still inspire a feud.

Margaret was not amused. It was just another potential flash point in an already precarious household. Eva stayed on weekends and some evenings. Sharon lived in during the week. Both Eva and Sharon were attentive and kind. Sharon read to my mother and got her to play word games. She stimulated her in ingenious ways we had never considered. She brought out the teacher in my mother, and it was beautiful to see.

One night Margaret was awakened at our home by a telephone call telling her that Sharon's brother had been murdered. Twenty-four years old, a cab driver in Brooklyn, a member of a religious, devoted family, murdered for a few bucks. It seemed impossibly unfair.

A few weeks later a woman called to interview me over the phone on the subject of love relationships in a family that has severe problems. How to split your loyalties. It sounded interesting. I had been on the "Today" show for four minutes right after the publication of the article, but I had never been interviewed by a newspaper or a magazine. I think I was atrocious. I went on and on and talked much too fast. I told the woman that I kept things from a man I was dating. I kept things like Sharon's brother being murdered.

She seemed appalled. "Why?" she asked.

"I am afraid to scare him away."

"But don't you think you owe him the honesty, the faith in his own ability to cut through the unimportant, and to understand that something like this, like this boy being murdered, is a horrible thing?"

I said that I was more afraid that he might think he was next.

I thought the interview was over. She went on. She seemed very determined and said I was making an "unfair judgment" about another person, who might very well be able to understand that I wasn't just an accident looking for a place to happen.

I told her that I felt most people must think of me as terribly — and, worse, contagiously — unlucky. I began to pour my heart out to this stranger on the phone, talking about my fears as I had never before addressed them.

I did keep a lot of the truth from many people I knew, because I felt very uncomfortable about it. Speaking about it made it real.

I was denying my mother's illness. But it was seeping in everywhere. I was making friends by it, writing about it, visiting my mother every Sunday, talking about almost nothing other than that with my sister.

By now, I allowed it to be the whetstone on which I sharpened my judgment of people. I resented people who borrowed trouble: friends at work with small fights with higher-ups. I resented anyone who complained about her family's interference in her life. And I judged people by their ability to deal with my problem — by whether they invited my mother and me over on a Sunday afternoon, approached us at the club at brunch on Sundays, called her or me or my sister to inquire about her condition or to take her out, went home with me on Sundays.

I was debating about writing a book. I had had several magazine offers and several calls from agents. I hadn't imagined having an agent. I felt as if I was kidding them on the phone, being very polite and worldly about my brilliant career, turning them down. But I hitched myself to one, and, as my father used to say, she was a "pip." She reminded me of my mother.

I was very unsure about writing a book. I called Priscilla, the former next-door terror, who had married nine years earlier, and asked her advice. She had three children, the first of whom, Alexander, was born with a red birthmark covering a large part of his head. At six months, the pulsing of the blood so close to the brain caused convulsions in the infant and left him, now eight, permanently undeveloped. He was beautiful, with vast eyes, but could do nothing for himself. He never even rolled over. Priscilla had told me that she was glad when I wrote my magazine piece — that she was tired of people ignoring diseases of the mind. I told her about the book offer.

Priscilla said, "Write it," in an angry tone that shocked me.

"Write it," she repeated. "When Allan [her husband] and I came home from the hospital that first time, we sat on the couch and cried. It was as if we sat there for weeks. We cried and held each other and cried some more. When I finally got off that damn couch and went to the bookstore, I found almost nothing. I was looking for a book on how to cope, just cope. I wasn't even looking for a cure. I just wanted to know how to live with this. The one book I did find was written by a man about his son who is dyslexic. The author goes on and on about his friends who are rock stars. I wish I had friends who are rock stars. But I don't. I'm just me, and Alexander is sick, and I live upstate, and

I don't know any damn rock stars, and I didn't know what the hell to do. Write the damn book, Marion," she said, crying into the phone.

My sister had a new boyfriend, Richard. They had met at Christmas when he was visiting New York from Australia with a friend of Margaret's who now lived in Sydney. Richard and Margaret had become close during his stay, and when he returned to Australia, they had corresponded. I had met him once; they seemed quite happy. By February they decided that he would move to the United States and live in the house in Douglaston.

Richard was devoted and intelligent and sensitive, and I liked him very, very much. Margaret was happy. She had a healthy, good-looking man to care for and be cared for by. I thought that things were getting a good deal better.

T. S. Eliot was wrong. April is not the cruelest month. March is. My grandfather died in March. My father died in March. I hate St. Patrick's Day. I hate March. I hate the weather. I hate the month.

A call from Richard tells me that Margaret has been rushed to the emergency room of the hospital. A terrible asthma attack. It is the fifth anniversary of my father's death, and my sister has gone into the hospital.

On my way out to the hospital I sing to myself a song with the lyrics "Break it to me gently. If you have to, tell me lies." I write in my notebook in a dense scribble, "My hair is not going white. I have no outward signs of tension."

Then, on the next line, in a worse scrawl, "Oh, yes, I do."

I visit my sister at the hospital that night. I am the most squeamish person I have ever met. Hospitals make me either throw up or pass out or both. Just the smell of them.

Scott goes with me to the hospital. We are standing in the room, and in the bed next to Margaret's is a small, huddled figure, partly hidden in the swirl of sheets. There is a family around a curled figure, and I am thinking of us at my father's bedside, and I feel very woozy and go out into the hall to look for a place to smoke a cigarette (which I do when I'm upset), and as I pass the bedside of the small figure I notice that it is a woman, and I hear her say, "What day is it, what time is it, what day is it?"

My sister is in a room with an Alzheimer's victim who has been brought in from a nursing home. My sister is in the hospital. She is exhausted, and my mother is driving her crazy at home. My sister has had an asthma attack that we all (including her doctor) believe may have been brought on by the stress and emotional trauma of my mother's illness, and she has been through the horrors of six hours in the emergency room and has landed in a room, five years to the day after my father died, in a bed next to a person who is asking what day it is.

I went berserk. I collared the doctor and I threatened insanity, in front of him, immediately. Of course I was being unsympathetic and selfish. But I thought it was about time. I had had it. The woman wasn't moved.

I never explained the problem. I didn't tell him about my mother and Margaret's stress. I just waved my arms around and yelled about having her moved. The staff must have thought I was crazy or selfish or both. I was not able, calmly, to start from the beginning and explain the causal factor. I didn't want to blame my mother. I didn't want to talk to strangers. I didn't seem to be getting anywhere. I don't think that the staff was familiar with Alzheimer's disease, which I did name as my mother's illness. I got a blank look from one nurse and a dull smile from another. I thought they should just understand. I was too frantic to be articulate.

Richard stayed with Margaret, in a chair next to the bed, every night. He helped her with her breathing exercises, talked positively about her future. I have never seen anyone so devoted to another human being. I will always love him for it. It was a remarkable display of what is possible with love. It was a remarkable lesson to me in how exhausted I was, how unable I was to be chipper and positive, and how someone coming in from outside was so much more able than I to provide hope and care.

Still March. Dr. Reisberg was writing a paper about that drug which he gave my mother at Christmas, the one that made her more agitated and no less confused. I was unhappy about the drug. Dr. Reisberg and I were having dinner in a Russian restaurant and were debating the value of the drug. It had helped some people. I felt cheated. Couldn't it have helped her, too?

As much control as I tried to exert over it in my conscious life, it was the disease that was exerting control over me, and it was in my subconscious that it struck back with a horrid vengeance. My nightmares were constant.

At the end of March I was awakened at four in the morning by my own shrieking. Then I started to cry. Soon, I was shaking, convulsing almost, and screaming. I was sweating, and I went into the bathroom, seeking the cool tiles of the floor. I was trying to get control. I sat down on the bathroom floor. Later, I wrote this in my journal.

My mother's illness is chasing down every bit of sanity I have left. My sanity is in bits, it is. Every scrap is being hunted and executed.

I dreamed she was doing ironing — her underwear. We were at someone's house but she was told to hang the clothes on a line because she's an idiot. I was showing her how to do it. She had underpants with large bloodstains. She didn't want to hang them. We had to leave. I left a man and other people at this house. I went home and started to laugh sickly and hysterically about how I could have just taken the car of this man and left him somewhere to care for this horrid woman. And yet I felt such kindness for her, such love, while she had been hanging the laundry and had noticed the bloodstains and had stopped and said, "I can't stand it, it's too horrible," and had put her head down and rolled it from side to side. "I can't stand it," she repeated. When we were home, someone came in carrying electric fans. He wants to get a look at her, I thought. He wants to see for himself. The man with the car called and I did not recognize his voice. "Who is this?" I asked. He was sweet and funny. He did not ask about his car or why I had left. He had, I knew, recognized the situation at the other house and, when not finding me there, had gone home. He was calling from home to say I should come over. I was on such good footing, I stupidly took my anger a step toward him and said in a most acerbic way that I'd have to call him back. He understood what was happening. I could tell by the tone of his voice. But he showed only slight annoyance and said all right. He is so good, I thought.

I went back to my mother. I was in the sun porch of the house in Douglaston. She was in her bedroom. There were cats perched everywhere, on the stairs, in the beds. I heard her rounding the corner into the porch. She had shaved her head into one thick stripe of hair down the middle of her skull and it was greasy. She smelled and she was filthy and the bones in her arms were sharp. She was thin and she was naked and she had a ghoulish, hollow, and determined look in her eyes when she stared at me. She was coming at me with her fingers out. She was quivering with sex. She was trying to touch me. She was shivering and smiling and reaching at me with long, bony fingers.

I put up my fists. "I just want to hit you and hit you," I said, and I kept swinging, but it was like under water, when there is no force. Nothing connected.

She kept coming toward me. She followed me into the bedroom and tried to touch me, tried to put her hand behind my head to kiss my lips, to touch her legs to mine. "Just a touch," she kept whispering, "to end this quivering. I am on the edge, just a touch," she said, with the hollow eyes and the smell.

That is when I started screaming. I sat on the bathroom floor, cursing her. I kept thinking that it was a search and destroy mission and that this time she was after sex, that she wanted me to have this image of her, naked and quivering, every time I even thought of sex. I sat on the floor and I shook and I wept and I didn't want to go back to the bed.

The next day I got drunk at lunch. I had too much to drink at dinner and went to sleep without reading. The next night I got drunk again. The entries in my journal are scribbled and thoughtless. I was thoughtless. Why is it that when we drink heavily we figure no one will notice? One friend tried to help me, tried to stick by me, realizing I was in terrible shape, but I tortured him by drinking and not talking, because I was afraid. It was three months before he spoke about it, let me know how angry he had been at my behavior, my drinking. Three months, unfortunately, of irreparable harm.

But then, by being what I considered a stoic, I was being a coward. I thought I was being a stoic by hiding in the bathroom, quietly getting drunk. When I emerged, I thought I was putting on my best face. I was blaming her, I was hiding from him, and no one benefited from it. I was allowing the disease to take more than one victim. I was looking for these horrendous experiences, and they were there.

I was willing not to cope; more than that, I was begging not to. Again. If it was happening again, it was going to happen forever, I figured. I was never going to get away from it. It was going to chase me down. She had been right, all those years ago: if something happened to her, it was going to destroy me, too.

A week before my birthday, I got a call at work.

"Hello, dear." I was stunned. It was my mother. She had stopped calling six months before. "How are you?"

"Fine, Ma. How are you?"

"Fine, thank you. I am calling because I want to know what you want for your birthday."

I was practically speechless. I hemmed and hawed. "Ah, is Margaret there?"

"Yes."

"Put her on the phone," I requested.

"Hi," said Margaret.

"What is this? Margy, did you put her up to it?" I asked.

"Swear to God, I didn't. She remembered all by herself and she's been up for hours, waiting to call you."

Good and bad. It's wonderful and touching that Allene remembered, but "up for hours"?

It was ten in the morning. She'd probably been sitting in my sister's bedroom since four, but Margaret wouldn't admit it when I pressed her about it. My older sister would protect me from myself if she possibly could.

On April 7, the actual day of my birthday, my mother called. "*Feliz cumpleaños,*" she said when I answered the phone.

"*Muchas gracias,*" I replied, and then, leading with my chin, as always, I said, "Hey, Ma, what language is that?"

"German."

"It's Spanish."

"No."

"French," she shot out into the phone.

"Uh-uh. No, Allene."

"Latin."

I was sorry, I really was, that I ever started this. It was so nice at the beginning of the conversation.

"Marion," she asked, "what did I get you for your birthday?"

This disease is a maniac. It goes through the life of the victim, ransacking the order of learning — dropping precious things it took years to acquire, forcing horrible new habits on its way. It hurtles through the helpless brain of the victim like electric shock through someone strapped down against her knowledge and will. She does know in the beginning. She knows and she hates it. Then it careers through the family, leaving them like loved ones standing beside those surgical straps, standing speechless and stunned by rage. We look to one another, we look at the victim, and we look away, for help. It goes on and on, and just when we can't stand another phase, we don't have to, because it's succeeded by another one — a worse phase, a more outrageous phase, a quieter phase, a sloppier phase, a more confused phase, a phase of hushed panic — seen in the eyes of the victim, seen by us. The one who knows best — the victim — about what is happening, loses the ability to tell us, the family, how to help. The ability to panic leaves the victim; it swarms over the family. As the victim forgets what is wrong, the family sees how it is, all very wrong.

I hate this disease.

Chapter 12

By the middle of April, Margaret had lost her privacy entirely. There was nearly always someone in the house and some question of management or scheduling to be handled. But despite the help, things were not working out. My mother would still pay attention to Margaret, despite my presence or that of Sharon or Eva. The questions, the constant questions, would be asked of Margaret after my mother had hunted her out with Sharon, Eva, or me in tow, through the house, in the bathroom, in the laundry room, or in her bedroom when Margaret was asleep.

"What day is it, Margaret?" "What time is it?" "When do I play tennis?" Over and over. "I have no clean clothes, no underwear." My mother would not take a shower, would not clean her ears, would put the same clothes on day after day. She insisted on wearing her fur coat every day, in the rain, when it got warm.

In April 1983, I stayed out at the house for a couple of days one week. I was in a room that was between my mother's bedroom and my sister's. Margaret and Richard were asleep. It was 6:15 a.m. when I heard the shower turn on and off and then on for a few minutes and then off again. I heard my mother's bedroom door open. Now it was 6:25, and it wasn't as if she had anywhere to go. But every morning, she got up at 6:15 and got dressed and went to Margaret's room and woke her up, and it was driving my sister into a hopeless rage. Margaret was beginning to hate the sight of her, and I understood.

There were chairs set up, here and there down the hall, blocking the way, one after another, like a set of barricades to Margaret's room. Each one had a sign: "Go back to bed." "Today is Tuesday." "Do not wake me until ten." My sister got home from work after one A.M.

Sometimes the signs deterred my mother. But not always. She would walk in on anyone in the shower. Richard was home all day. He leased a computer and was working as a commodities trader in a room he had set up as an office. He liked the freedom of working at home on his own schedule. Sometimes he would shower in the middle of the day. When my mother heard any noise, she tracked it down like a ray. The shower was a perfect target. She had walked in on Richard a dozen times. She would just look at him and ask what day it was. We tried to remember to lock the doors, but if we forgot, just once, there she was.

It was 6:25. She was coming out her bedroom door and heading, I was sure, for Margaret. I leaped out of bed; she was standing in the hall, shower cap, like a helmet, halfway across her eyeballs. She was naked except for a garter belt, and the cap was not wet. I was sure she had never got in the shower.

"Where are you going?" I whispered, almost giggling at her get-up.

She dipped her shoulder and faked left and went right, under my arm, which was on the banister, and said, "No stockings, no stockings, I haven't got any stockings." In rhythm, just like that. Like the White Rabbit late for a very important date, she dashed down the stairs, and I heard her do a lap around the living room. I was standing at the top of the stairs, in some form of slight shock, when I saw her come back up the stairs, straight at me. Her garter snaps were flapping up and down. She knocked into me, I banged into the wall, and she leaped over the threshold of her bedroom and slammed the door. When I went in, she was under the covers in her bed, eyes shut, with the shower cap still slammed down on her head.

"Okay, all right, what's going on here?" I said to her, standing over her bed. I was laughing. What else was I going to do? Cry? It was absurd. The scene was absurd.

"I'm sleeping."

The next night I was to take her to dinner. I told her to take a shower.

"I won't wash my hair," she said defiantly.

It was a common response. She hated to wash her hair. I don't know why. She was always rushing. Everything had to be done quickly. She seemed desperately afraid of missing something. She would plot and plot to be able to cut a second off any procedure. But it wasn't as if she had a great deal to do. Actually she was grasping at any recognizable event, probably, desperately trying to hold on to it.

"Please wash your hair," I said.

"No."

"Then we're not going to dinner."

"Marion, why? Why aren't we going to dinner. Oh, please."

"Allene, just wash your hair, please. We don't have to be there for an hour and a half."

"I don't have time."

It went on and on. I waited and heard the water running. I was reading. Then when she was finished I got into my shower. Cold water. More cold water. The hot water heater frequently shut itself off. It had been happening all my life. It had to be fiddled with and I was in no mood to coax it — and it takes hours for the water to heat.

I was furious. But I showered.

I went in to see her progress. I was really in a rage about the water. It was stupid, but despite what I read, anger is not a gun; it's a cannon, and you can't just point it and fire it. At least, I tried not to, at her. I searched for other places to let it off.

I was pacing around her bathroom. She was setting her hair. It wasn't clean. She hadn't washed it.

"What's wrong?" she asked me.

"No hot water. Dammit. Did you have hot water?"

"Oh, yes."

"You did?"

"Oh, yes."

I looked in the shower. I don't know why, but I looked at the shower itself. It has elaborate fixtures, including six broad nozzles with pinhole openings lining the tiled walls, and a tester at the foot. I spun one of the heavy porcelain nozzles. Cold.

"You had hot water?"

"Oh, yes," she said, rolling a clump of hair.

"Are you sure?"

"Oh, yes."

"Wait a minute, why the hell am I asking you? You don't know what you're talking about. You don't know what day it is. What am I doing?"

What the hell was I doing? It was a very cruel thing to say.

But she laughed and shook her head, like a parent whose child does some stupid inexplicable thing, and she kept rolling her hair and shaking her head and laughing to herself, and for a moment I was the kid with her fist through a wall and she was the parent who found me and she was laughing at my plain dumb anger. And for a moment she was my mother again. Because of my cruelty.

. . .

There were signs everywhere. We had become accustomed to them. We had started in her bedroom, labeling the drawers — "Underwear," "Slips." What once had been a symmetrical bedroom — two beds, over each a portrait of a daughter, two dressers, two nightstands, each with a matching lamp — now was cluttered with signs. Some said, "We love you," but most had to do with the day of the week, the directions for the shower, the contents of a drawer.

Soon they spread. The hall outside Allene's bedroom was a freeway of billboards. "Go back to sleep," one read. "Do not go into Margaret's room," said another. "Do not go out alone," on the doors downstairs. "This time is right," on her clock. "Put butter in pan before egg," over the stove. Up they went as we found the need, but we were always one sign behind and would realize that only when the shoes were in the shower or when the surviving cats gained five pounds each. Up would go another sign.

"The cats have been fed." "Shoes in the closet." "Do not open," on the windows downstairs. "Do not use as an ashtray," on her soap dish. The house looked crazy, littered with signs, some old, some new. Margaret's room was the only rectangular space without a sign, but there was one on the outside of her door. It just said, "No."

The signs worked. They kept Allene out of trouble. They kept her in bed, away from the big windows, off the balcony at the front of the house, out of the basement.

Alzheimer's victims pace. They seem to need no sleep. But as long as she could read, she could be deterred. Margaret needed sleep, and the only way she could get it was by knowing that Allene was out of trouble.

It did not have the look of a happy house. It was not a happy place to be.

The stove might seem an obvious danger area, but my

mother never cooked unless there was someone with her, unless someone actually made her cook. She would simply eat anything she could get her hands on while standing in front of the refrigerator. If she had slipped away from you for a moment, it was an easy guess that you would find her, one hand dipped into something, another wiping something on her shirt, in front of the fridge, as seemingly engrossed as she would be, moments later, in front of the television. Eating wasn't interesting — certainly not enough to make her cook — but it was something to do. Once, Margaret came home at one A.M. and opened the front door to an overpowering smell of gas. My mother probably had been trying to light a cigarette and had lost her matches. We had taken the lighters away, because I had seen her try to light the gas jets with a lighter and was afraid it would blow up in her hand. She couldn't manage the push button that ignited the gas from the jet. Aged fifty-four, she couldn't push a button after spinning a dial. But she could still spin the dial.

Margaret smelled the gas, ran to the stove, and found one jet streaming gas. She turned it off and as she opened the back door to get fresh air, she burst into tears.

Soon there was another incident with the gas. Everyone was asleep when Margaret again came home at one in the morning and found that a gas jet had been spun open. After the first incident we had looked into getting locks for the gas dials, but it had too soon become apparent that the entire kitchen was a hazard, like the rest of the house. Now there were were signs all over the kitchen, too. Every window, every plastic bag, looked like a weapon; there was danger in every item. That was the way we thought. Everything had to be reassessed for its potential harm.

And as we — as I would learn to say — chewed more gum and plugged more holes, my mother continued to career through her remaining awareness. She would refuse to use a spatula, turning a fried egg with her hands if you looked away for a second, and when the egg broke and ran down her wrists, she would gaze at the pain from the heat, upset by the mess and ashamed by her confusion.

The kitchen became a war zone.

"Mom, use a knife, please."

"A knife?" she repeats. She quickly scans the area and doesn't see one. She continues what she is doing.

My mother is holding an unwrapped stick of butter in her fist. It is oozing between her fingers and out either end of her grasp. She is clenching the butter and rubbing one end against a dry piece of cold toast. We are alone in the kitchen.

"A knife, yeah, please. A knife for the butter, Ma."

"What else is wrong with me? What else would you like to correct?" she asks me. "What else do I do wrong? Oh, leave me alone."

She slaps the stick of butter against the counter and it stays there, marks from her fingers and hand circling it. She leaves the kitchen.

I look at the floor. My feeling is of anger that is tired, very, very tired. I'm tired of it, she's tired of it, but it is always there. It is more than table manners. It is more than the defiance we shared when Grandma would quote Emily Post to "the girls" — my mother, my sister, and me.

This is madness, I think. "This is madness," I say out loud.

But I know better. This is Alzheimer's disease.

The behavioral concomitants were tripling and tripping over one another. Smoking, for instance, became a real issue. She would wake Margaret up, she would call a friend, she would stop people in the street, she would get out the door, away from the attendants — she would do anything to get a cigarette. When she was smoking, she seemed to be doing something normal. It was an outward sign that she was in control. And she smoked constantly. The smoking didn't bother me if I could keep it under control, I thought, but doling out one cigarette an hour to your mother, who couldn't remember that she had just smoked one and wore you down with "Can I have another cigarette" until you gave her one and she left it burning on the couch was a phenomenon that was strange at first but became familiar.

Margaret's life was scheduled around keeping one step ahead of Allene. My sister made hair appointments, tennis dates, movie dates, bowling appointments, for our mother. Allene could go out. If completely attended, she could participate in social activities, asking questions all the while, but hitting the ball back on a court during a game of tennis, like a ball machine, or rolling the bowling ball endlessly down the alley. She was only repetitive and confused. Socially, she was annoying, but she was hardly inept. Given an activity, she'd do it until it was over. Handed a box of buttons to sort, she'd sit all day. If you hit her a tennis ball, she'd slam it back to you, over and over and over, until you walked off the court and she followed, mechanically, asking questions over and over. She could not keep score, but she could smash an overhead, rack up a strike, and then you had to change her to the other side of the court or lead her from the alley. She could play tennis, she could bowl, but she couldn't manage the details of the game. She could do practically anything — except remember.

The phone with automatic dialing became her best friend, unfortunately. My mother started calling directory assistance somewhere in the neighborhood of eighty times a day to ask what time it was, what day it was. Margaret protested the first bill — $176. Triple the previous month's. We couldn't figure out the charge. And then one day Margaret heard her on the phone ask what day it was, and then a few minutes later, heard her do it again.

I was at work. Margaret was on the phone. I could tell without even a hello on the other end, because she was gearing up for a large wail, and my sister always inhales before she cries. I had heard a lot of it by this time. She would call me when she was depressed and exhausted. She would let out in a rush a great many things she didn't really mean — how she couldn't stand another minute, another question — and then she would become composed and stop crying and we would make some alteration, make a decision to help her.

This time Margaret wanted to talk about locking the phones. We could not afford the bills. And there was one more thing. Some of my mother's "friends" had started calling Margaret and complaining that Allene was harassing them at work, making them feel "guilty" by calling and asking when she was scheduled to see them when, in fact, she wasn't scheduled to see them at all. She wanted them to take her to church or go bowling or play tennis. Sometimes she just wanted to know the time of day.

And so we agreed that we should lock the phones, and Margaret went to the hardware store.

Later that afternoon I got another call from Margaret. Again, she was crying. But this time there was anger in her voice. "Do you know what it's like," she asked, "do you have any idea what it is like to lock a phone in front of your mother and have her stand there and then reach up and put her fingers on the small lock and look at you and just say, just say, 'Why are you doing this to me?' "

No, I didn't have any idea and I got only an inkling when I went there two days later on Sunday and my mother asked me over and over and over again why Margaret had locked the phones. "Why did Margaret lock the phones?"

"Because she had to, Allene."

"Why?"

"Because you were making too many calls to the operator and we can't afford it."

Why did Margaret lock the phones? Why?

"Please unlock them. Please. I promise I won't call anybody," she said, clutching my forearm with one hand and touching the phone with the other.

"Then why the hell do you want them unlocked?" I snapped.

Logic is a horrible, unwanted companion. Logic said that she was fifty-four and fine. Logic said that logic was understood. Logic had no and has no place in the climate of this type of illness. Logic said that she wanted them unlocked because the lock meant that she was not competent to be left alone with a phone, that she was losing more ground, and that we were filling that space with restrictions. Logic said I could never look her in the eyes and be so mean. So much for logic.

At the end of April I hung up on my friend Tracy. She was at home, sick with a cold, and called me at work. Tracy had had a touch-and-go relationship with her older sister for years, and it recently had developed into a warm and honest friendship. I think we all knew it would eventually, and it was nice to see it. But when she called and wanted to tell me "how very important it is that sisters be close to one another," I didn't want to hear about it.

Tracy had been with me to visit my mother. She had packed me back onto the train at midnight more than once when I was incompetent and berserk and confused.

My relationship with Margaret was exceedingly strained, and not through any fault of our own, I thought; I resented the fact that we fought. It wasn't a good, clean fight, ever. It never had the chance to be over an idea or a blouse; it was always, without fail, about Mommy, her care, the expense, the hours put in, which my sister always went into and came out of better than I did. I didn't live in the house, so I lived with the huge guilt of an absentee daughter. My sister wanted to live in the house. It is large and lovely, and Richard was there, and nearly every argument would come down to that. I wished with all my heart that someday we could just fight like two cats over something other than my mother.

It occurred to me, then, that we really had been fighting about Allene all our lives, that Margaret and I had never agreed about her. I loved her, and Margaret preferred to remain aloof, showing no feeling toward her, except the feeling that she should do the right thing — show up for a birthday, for Christmas, because of family obligation. She was caring for her now because of family obligation, whereas I was hurting, and was not taking very good care of her, because of love. Very different. Absolutely different.

So when Tracy started telling me about the closeness of sisters, I got mad. She said, "You know, there have been so many times — I know it hasn't been easy — when you've been able to take things in stride and just say, 'Oh, let's have a beer,' but you're not doing that now."

"Sometimes I take it all in stride," I said, "but other times I get angry and I get resentful and I've just had it, okay?" and I hung up.

Tracy was completely within her rights. And I truly was happy about her new friendship with her sister. I was wallowing in grief without knowing it. I had been preparing myself for a long time for my mother's death in inches, and as it came nearer, showing itself to us in these hideous lapses of her mind, I became more and more panicky. I was suffering from some sort of emotional blindness; it was difficult if not impossible to see past it, to see that there was a future, no matter how close. This blindness, like nausea, was all-consuming. It was impossible to think about ever eating again; it was impossible to think about others' feelings. If I accepted that my mother was going to die, then I accepted that I could handle it. If I could handle it, I wanted it right away, not in little pieces like this, shreds, really, of her mind falling away right before me. Since it was not to be immediate, I stopped accepting it. She's not going to die. She's going to linger. It was like going to a funeral — every day.

Different friends had different approaches. Tracy was right in refusing to let me ignore the rest of the world, and I probably gave her the hardest fight, but she stuck right to it. Marianne always tried humor, like a message she left on my recording machine:

> I called to complain. Do you know what they are doing with M & M packages now? They are making them harder to open. Do you have some contact with the company? Where are you? I'll be here all night, so call me later. Oh, are you at your Alzheimer's meeting tonight? Is this Wednesday? What day is it? What time is it? Who have I called? [Laughter.] I'm sorry. Hope you had a nice time. Call me if you need to.

She got a lot of calls from me late on Wednesday nights. I was, almost without exception, depressed on Wednesdays, after my group, but it was a depression with a purpose, a sadness with a focus, not an elusive fear or unattended mourning. It was all right to care, and I did, then. Through the therapy, however, I had learned that it was all right to care, always, as long as I didn't do damage to myself.

My friendships were as varied as my anger.

One day my mother called me Myra. Then she called me Pat and then Margaret. It came out like rapid shots — "Myra, ah, Pat, Margaret" — followed by a stare of dismay, of nonrecognition, of frustration.

I knew all about this. I had learned about it in my Alzheimer's group. But knowing about it did not prepare me for the first time she was confused about my name. Next, I was told, she would be confused about my identity. Then she would not know who I was.

I knew better than to get angry, but I got angry. I care for her emotionally and physically, and she forgets my name? My Alzheimer's training told me that it was the disease that was making the person forget my name. My mother was not forgetting my name; it was the disease. I got angry anyway. I wish I could say I got angry with the disease, but I got angry with her. Scott was there, but it didn't stop me from losing my temper.

"Who is Myra, Mom?"

No answer. We didn't know anyone named Myra.

"Who is Myra?" I asked again, in anger. "Not me. Not me, Ma. I'm not Myra. I know who Pat is, and I'm not Pat. I'm not Margaret, Ma. I'm Marion, your younger daughter. Marion, Ma. Marion, goddammit."

By this time my mother had forgotten saying anything, so she stared at me, at my expression of anger, of rage, of grief. Frustration looking at anger and dismay. Scott looked at us in despair and impotence. What could he do? Who was wrong? What was wrong? What wasn't wrong? It was all wrong. She was too young; she was too sick. I was too mad; he was too hurt. I did this every time I got angry — I condensed it, zooming right back to the start: it was wrong, all wrong from the start. I looked at him. I looked at her. It was awful. It was like our being chained to each other and tossed in the water. No one could swim.

I backed away, Scott retreated with me, and my mother went off in another direction. I was embarrassed in front of my friend, hurt for myself, and in anguish over being so mean to my mother. Scott put his arm around me, called me "Mar," as he often did, and then, a few steps later, said,

"You're not handling this very well, Mar." An innocent but concerned thing to say. He was right. He was certainly my closest friend. He had to say something. I said nothing, but later that night I wrote the following in my journal:

> People tell me that I am not handling this well. I wonder what "well" is. Happy, perhaps? Gleeful to be of any service? I resent so very deeply when they criticize my reactions. I deeply resent Scott telling me that I cannot stand to sit through dinner with my mother, that I shouldn't yell. That may be, but I get through it, don't I? I don't mean to be mean or cruel or anything other than, perhaps, defensive. And he says I am not handling it. I don't remember ever crying in front of him or walking out.
> My mother's disease was out of the blue and I am leveled by it. Even now, after five years of it, I feel that it is out of the blue. An anger is supposed to cause a war, generate a punch, stop a life. I am angered into sleep and sloth. I am angered to the point of passivity.

Inaction, like hanging up on Tracy. Giving up instead of listening or thinking about others, thinking about life and how it goes on. I smoked again, a lot. I drank too much. I slept too much. I ignored everything, and I hurt too much. I wanted to call back when I hung up on Tracy, but I couldn't.

I was also jealous, I now realize, that she was just coming into her relationship with her sister. A nice, clean slate, I thought. I was jealous, and also the next day I was to move my mother's furniture from her home, out from under her, into an apartment Margaret and I had bought. I felt, I suppose, some form, some undiagnosed, unspecified form, of righteous indignation about the whole thing.

It was just the beginning of May. The apartment Margaret had found was less than a mile from the house in Douglaston. We had finally realized that the house was too big and keeping her there too dangerous and too difficult for even the most conscientious caretaker. She needed twenty-four-hour, seven-day-a-week supervision and care. We were borrowing more money than I had ever seen, to be paid back after the year 2000 at a rate that would make the money returned more than three times what we were borrowing, to put our mother out of the house she loved.

We live in a country that does not believe in preventive medicine; in a country where someone suffering from a condition without a cure is without medical reimbursement. My mother suffers from a disease that requires that she have constant care, that she be constantly watched lest she do herself harm — by swallowing a poison, walking into the snow without a coat, getting lost. Another person is her life line, her life-support machine.

We have a wonderful, sensitive lawyer, who over the past several years has changed his practice so that it is now devoted almost solely to problems of the Alzheimer's patient. He and his partner have pioneered programs to care for the living but incapable person. Instead of life insurance, to be paid to the family at the death of a loved one, Peter Strauss and his partner, Robert Wolf, try to get people to manage their funds for the proper care of the living. They helped Margaret and me set up a system whereby my mother would live outside the home in a cooperative apartment so that when she died the sale of the apartment might cover some of the cost of her care.

The first time I met Peter, we cried together as he told me about a man, a victim of Alzheimer's, who was literally huddling in the past; he kept himself all curled up, even when walking. He thought he was back in a concentration camp, where he had spent his young adulthood. The first time the man was in Peter's office, he leaped out of his chair and threw himself under the desk when the secretary entered. Since our first meeting, Peter has been added to the family my sister and I accept as we lose Allene.

After the move, Peter figured that the cost to us, including the apartment rent, would be $4000 a month, all of which was totally nonreimbursible. The attendants alone cost $420 a week. The cost of maintenance of the apartment for one month was less than we paid for my mother's attendants for a week. All of her assets were transferred early in the course of her disease into a trust to pay for her care, and that, plus the income that Margaret and I managed to contribute, maintained her as long as possible. At the time of the move, she was legally destitute. The trust was in our name, with the provision that it go just for her care; in other words, we transferred her money to us to be spent only on her. Margaret and I kept the house, and Margaret continued to live there.

Two years after a transfer of this sort, a family may apply for medical assistance from the government. There is no guarantee that it will be granted, and such transfers are heavily reviewed. Medicaid may, at some point, pay for home care, but getting it to do so is a very difficult process, which I was later to learn.

Simply put, Medicaid is for the poor and Medicare for the old. At fifty-four, and with some funds, my mother was neither, so we, like other middle-income families, were left to fend for ourselves until we become dependents of the state.

We did not consider a nursing home; we could not justify it. The average age of the nursing home resident in this country is over eighty. The average cost of a home is $36,000 a year, which would be picked up by the government once my mother's assets were used up, but we couldn't stand the idea. We decided to do everything else before even considering such placement.

The house in Douglaston became the only hedge Margaret and I had against the future. We borrowed against it to pay for my mother's care, knowing that we probably would go broke and my mother would have to go into a home. But we decided to take the gamble and hope for something — anything — to happen. Maybe, we thought, we could find a roommate for her and then another and set up a house, owned by several families, with a couple of live-in companions. We worked out the project with Peter, and it gave us hope.

Alzheimer's patients at my mother's stage need very little if any medical care. She needed only to be given her medication once a day. Other than that, she needed aid and she needed to be watched. Therefore, one companion could care for several people if they were at the same stage. We thought we'd pioneer the field. We had such tremendous hope for the project. But we kept being told that it would be cheaper, still, to put her in a home, where she would be fully covered by Medicaid. That is the system we have built in this country. That is the health care we provide at the end of a prosperous life.

We came to hope that if our plan didn't work, my mother would die before we ran out of money, before we had to place her in a home. It was not only the worst feeling I had ever contemplated but it was also unrealistic. There was no reason to believe that she would die soon.

At the time we knew that she might stay at the confused stage for three or four more years before she moved into a demented phase, a phase of severe incompetence, of incontinence, possible loss of speech, total loss of recognition. I hoped she would die soon, because I knew that she was still aware enough of her illness to be unhappy. I hoped that she would die soon, because the economics of the situation made me feel that way.

My ethics had taken a turn I had never anticipated.

On April 27, aided by my mother's friend Lette and five large and wonderful friends of mine, I moved my mother.

I was nervous. Margaret asked to be excused from the exercise. She was exhausted, and she had done all the initial work on the apartment: hanging draperies, getting the painters, filling the refrigerator, measuring for the rug. I stopped at Lette's and had a drink first and then we proceeded, a somber group, to the house. My old friend Jimmy was one of the group. He lived across from Lette and Tom and up the street from the school my mother attended as a girl. Jimmy was my favorite mid-thirties Peter Pan; he could rig a boat and catch a fish with the gutsy enthusiasm of Tom Sawyer and could usually talk about anything. He said he just wanted to move her and get it over with and "talk about it later." He looked as if someone had died.

My mother was supposed to be out with a friend. I walked in with my group and we started lifting a table, the couches, and I noticed Lette stop for a moment and look to her right and then at me, and I looked at her and then I looked to my right, and there was my mother. In a room full of young men hoisting a table bought on her honeymoon, my mother looked at Lette and asked, "When are we bowling again?"

I left the room.

There was nothing left. No recognition, no interest, just an inkling, an association with Lette and bowling, and nothing more. My dismay was total. My guilt gave way to anguish, and three days later we moved the things from her bedroom and then we moved her.

It was a terrible plot. The day before the move, Lisa called Margaret and said, "I can't let you do it." She wasn't talking about letting us move Allene. She was talking about letting us do it alone.

We had been getting hang-up calls from people — neighbors, I suppose — who criticized "moving your mother" and then hung up. We knew Lisa wasn't calling to criticize.

Lisa volunteered to take my mother out to dinner and then take her to the new apartment. She said she couldn't let us be the ones to take her there. I first had to get my mother's purse and put the new keys on her chain and remove all the old ones. As I stood in my old bedroom with my mother's purse stuffed under my sweatshirt (getting it away from her required some quick work, because she almost never let go of it; it seemed to be her touchstone of reality, as if sifting through it and seeing the objects within meant she was fine), I started to think about what we were doing. We were tricking her. We were playing to the disease. I exchanged the keys and I felt like a heel.

Lisa and Allene went out to dinner. Richard and I dashed over to the apartment and transformed it into an exact replica of the house: the position of the couches, the pictures on the wall. But we put only one of the two beds from the master bedroom into her new bedroom, and that made me cry. One bed. My parents had always slept in two identical beds, next to each other.

Richard and I stacked college yearbooks and arranged lingerie. I moved the drawers — all labeled — full, as they were before, so that they would look the same to her when she opened them.

When Lisa brought my mother to the apartment, Eva was there in front of the television, as always; the refrigerator was full; and Mommy was a little confused. But Lisa said, "Allene, you've been staying here for a few weeks. The roof fell in at the house [I will always think that choice of words particularly appropriate] and you've been living here since then. You will be here until it's fixed. Now show me around."

And Allene, ever cautious of making a mistake, ever wary of doing the wrong thing, even then able to wing it like a trooper, took a look at all sides and said, "Well, this is the living room . . ."

Using her confusion, we had played a trick. It worked, and she settled in.

The day before the move was my last day at the *New York Times*. I was sad but relieved. I hadn't found a niche there, and I wanted to try something else.

The day before that, Thursday, I had gone out to dinner and had seen Laurence Olivier in the restaurant. He was eating two spoonfuls of caviar on a plate and gingerly squeezing a lemon over them. He sat erect as an owl and he moved like a swan. He was with his wife and a woman who was eating fresh vegetables with her fingers. I couldn't take my eyes from her. She didn't look the way my mother did when she ate with her hands.

Saturday we moved my mother. Sunday Richard and I visited and took her out to lunch. She asked me again and again why she was living in an apartment, when she could go "home." I felt very guilty and very sad.

Several months earlier I had received an invitation to speak at a conference on bereavement. All of a sudden it was here, two days after the move. My subject was "Grieving Before the Funeral." I had never made a speech before and I had no idea why I had been invited to make this one. I was nervous and I had written nothing out. On the way uptown I jotted a few notes.

There were several hundred people in the audience. When I was asked to sit at the front at the speakers' table, it suddenly became painfully clear to me that I was to make a real speech. I was told to try to hold it to twenty minutes. Twenty minutes? There was no way I could speak about grief for twenty minutes. I didn't know a thing about it, I thought.

The first speaker, Dr. Avery D. Weisman, professor of psychiatry at Harvard, was talking about dealing with an "appropriate death," a death that you can live with, and he said that the three necessary characteristics for a "good bereavement" are compassion (a feeling for someone without feeling their feelings), courage, and a sense of timeliness. "Theoretically," he said, "there ought to be a death that's right on time."

He explained that in cases of long-term illness, the family starts to grieve the moment the diagnosis is made. In such cases, death is not an end but a stage.

Grieving. I was grieving, but I thought it was a quicksand emotion, down and out and gone forever. Dr. Weisman was saying that grieving is a process. Not static, but with motion. And not eternal.

"My name is Marion Roach, and when I first was asked to speak here, I couldn't understand it. I thought, Why me? I certainly don't know anything about grief.

"But now, I think I do."

I talked about how in the beginning we had set up a "buddy system" for my mother that had become a life-support system. I talked about the lack of moral guidance when a parent is diminishing before you, the resentment, the guilt. I explained how, as I moved through these stages, I had learned a great deal about grief.

My heart was pounding so that I could hear it in my voice, clogging my words at regular intervals. And then I thought of my favorite writer, Emily Dickinson, and I quoted from memory the last four lines of my favorite poem of hers. It begins with "After great pain, a formal feeling comes," and ends with these lines:

> This is the Hour of Lead —
> Remembered, if outlived,
> As Freezing persons recollect the Snow —
> First Chill, then Stupor, then the letting go —

I was letting go. I looked up and realized that I had spoken for fifteen minutes, and then I looked into the audience and saw that a lot of people were crying. When I was finished, people stood in line to talk with me, to kiss me, to hold my hand, and for the first time in four years I knew that I was going to be all right. Just knowing that it was a process —

this grief — a system, not a random, haphazard, inexplicable force, but something, horrible as it was, that people studied, that people discussed as an entity, somehow I knew that I wasn't going along for the ride on the tail of this disease. And neither was Margaret.

A week later I went to my high school tenth reunion. There had been twenty-four girls in the class. Eighteen showed up. Only one other than I had yet to be married. Several were pregnant. Most had children. I sat at a table with Ellen, who had two children; Renée, who had just had her first; Carin, who was divorced; and Claudia, who was eight months pregnant. Claudia was a dentist, married to a doctor. She was living in the Midwest and had come in to see her parents before the birth and to attend the reunion.

She told us that she had been standing in the shower earlier that evening when there was a knock on the door. Her mother had asked if she could come in. Once inside the room, she had said, "Can I see?" She wanted to see Claudia pregnant. They swept back the shower curtain and looked, together, at the wonder.

The Tin Man was right about when you know you have a heart. These things touched me deeply. To me, it was an entirely beautiful image. It was one of the things I knew I would never know.

I called my mother the next morning and asked her if she had received the plant I sent her for Mother's Day.

"Ah, well," she said, stammering a bit, "every day is Mother's Day."

I chuckled. "You bet. But did you get the plant, Allene?"

Another hesitation. "Yes."

"Good," I said, but I was suspicious. Just suspicious. Either she didn't get it or she didn't know what I was talking about and she was stalling, and I wanted to know which. Why? Because I was angry all the time, and if the florist hadn't delivered it, good, because I could call up and scream, and if I was pursuing it only to find that she was as confused as I knew she was, then I was a fool.

Hesitation. "It's very pretty."

She was still marvelously able to tap-dance her way through uncomfortable situations, given the right circumstances and a lack of confrontation. But when I went out the next day and stupidly asked again, she didn't know where she had gotten the plant that was in her living room.

My mother still loved being with people. She was armed with her date book, to which she would refer hundreds of times a day, to make her aware — for a moment — of the date. With another person at her side, she could go for an afternoon walk or a meal out, looking beautiful and simply being repetitive. Some people found it less upsetting than others. A few of her friends seemed absolutely at ease with her and liked to have us come over to watch television or have a weekend lunch. One was Lette.

Her daughter was getting married in May and she wanted me to bring my mother for as long or short a time as I felt Allene would be comfortable. My mother had it written in her date book and talked about nothing else for the week before the celebration. It was a social situation that I judged her able to handle. I figured that we would stay an hour. The ceremony was private. I knew that Allene would ask the same questions over and over, but I knew, too, that she enjoyed her time at Lette and Tom's, and that made me happy. She smiled a lot when she was there. She told the few, same stories over and over about the house they lived in and going to school with Lette, and she smiled when people laughed at them.

I knew she'd enjoy the wedding, yet I was terribly nervous in the car before picking her up. I remember pulling over to the side of the road when I got to Douglaston and talking to myself, just smoothing out the wrinkles of my nervousness. And then thinking that there was nothing to fear. I slipped in an Ella Fitzgerald tape and drove myself along the water before picking her up, listening to some of our favorite songs. It would be a tough day, I knew, but I expected that. There was nothing for me to do now but relax.

She was dressed and ready, except that her dress was askew and the nails on one hand were polished, but not on the other. I suggested we apply some more polish.

"No," she said and started for the door.

"Allene, come on."

"No." Her voice was like sandpaper. She was pacing. She wanted out then and there, and it was trickery that won. I got her to take off her shoes and hid them long enough for me to get the nails polished, and then we left.

We were standing outside Lette and Tom's. "So what did you do today?" I asked her.

She started for the door, a look of determination on her face, her jaw thrust out, grinding her teeth slowly, as she did when really trying to concentrate, when she looked her most demented. She's not listening, I thought. She was marching into that party and she was going to be with people and she had been talking about it for a week — almost nothing but that.

She flipped her head to my side and I saw that the look of vengeance had passed. "I had sex." She opened the door and marched in.

I was lagging behind. I was stunned.

But this was not the time to discuss it. She was through the door and heading directly for Lette. Lette has the most positive nature. She didn't flinch. She hugged my mother and waved me away with her hand.

I went to the bar and started talking with someone and then was walking back to her when I saw Allene turn to the mother of the groom — she had never met her before — and say something in a very animated way, and I saw the wedding corsage dip and the woman look inquiringly into my mother's face and I thought, Oh, my God, she's telling her that she had sex today.

On my way back to my mother I picked something from the buffet table and popped it into my mouth. It stuck. Stupidly, I hid my problem from the people at the party. I went upstairs and tried everything I could to get the thing dislodged. I was embarrassed. I couldn't bring myself to go downstairs and cause more trouble. My mother, I thought, was trouble enough. I didn't realize it, but I was upstairs for two hours, and when I came down, Lette told me that someone had taken my mother home. The people at the party figured I had gone across the street to see friends; they never suspected I had been upstairs. I called my mother. She was fine.

I got in the car and drove by myself to Manhattan, spitting up into a cup the entire way. I couldn't swallow. Every time I did, it came back up. I went to the emergency room. It was two A.M. After several hours of young residents rubbing sleep from their eyes while taking x rays, telling me that, yes, indeed, something was there, and then finally shoving a thick tube down my throat and pushing whatever it was into my stomach, they let me go. What they didn't realize was that somehow my esophagus had gotten punctured. The x rays showed a hole through which air escaped into my throat, and seven of them missed it. They let me walk out.

Two days later, a doctor called. "Is this Marion Roach?" she asked.

I was in bed with an extremely sore throat and was feeling lousy. "Yes," I mumbled.

"I have reviewed your x rays from this morning."

The x rays were then two days old.

"You are in terrible danger; you have to come right back."

I told her that I would never come back there and that

she was very irresponsible to say such a thing to me. I told her to call my doctor immediately. She did, and five minutes later my internist called and told me to get to a hospital right away.

I spent seven days in Doctors' Hospital, the first five with the warning that I not so much as swallow my own saliva. If I had a hole, I was told, there was a chance of a heart and lung infection. They would monitor me for five days, with no food, only heavy intravenous antibiotics, and then the decision would be made as to whether to operate.

The doctor said that I might die. He asked me about my family. He said he had read my article about my mother. I just kept nodding and thinking about being that sick; how it had happened in an instant. He asked me if I had any other family.

My sister was away at a newspaper conference in Washington. Richard was with her. They came back immediately. It was when my sister walked into the room that I began to feel real fear. It had seemed that nothing could happen to me with no family around, but with her — virtually my entire family, Margaret — standing there, looking scared but sounding like the voice of confidence, I fell apart.

When I got out after a week without the operation, "miraculously lucky," according to the doctor, I began to review the event with a startled eye. Sex. Could she be having sex? Did it matter?

"Of course it matters," I insisted.

"Why does this bother you so much, Marion?"

I was at my support group the week after getting out of the hospital. I had not seen my mother since the wedding reception. I was afraid to. Guilt. Grief. Sadness. Despair. Now fear. Now I was afraid of her.

I thought I had learned to manage the other ones. But fear? Things just seemed to go wrong when we were together. Now I thought I was going to die if I saw her.

"Can't you just talk about it with her?" Emma asked.

"Apparently not," I said with a sarcasm that had become entirely too familiar. "The last time I did, I stuffed a leg of lamb down my throat." Everyone laughed a little, and I did too, until I started to cry.

If my mother was having sex, was it any of my business? Well, sure it was, because I wouldn't allow her to be hurt by anyone, and I would chop up anyone who was taking advantage of her. But what if it was a pleasurable experience for her? I still did not want to relinquish any aspect of the mother-daughter relationship. I wanted to remain the child, and I did not want to know anything about an affair, anything about sex. I wanted to be naïve on that subject. Then, I thought, I was leaving alone an issue in her life; I was giving her some privacy, which is what children are supposed to do.

If it weren't for her illness, I wouldn't have known about it, because she never intended that I know, and I kept trying to tell myself that I should just let it slide.

Sex. I didn't want to know any more. I knew everything about my mother's brain. I knew that inside, behind the eyes and skull, it was beginning to look as if someone had blown holes in it, at close range, with a shotgun. I knew about her ovaries, her heart; I had seen her medical records. I had handled, during the move, letters I was never meant to see; I had opened unpaid bills, of which she would have been ashamed; I had seen her handwriting become sprawling and seen her fingers turn yellow from cigarettes; I had put expandable sections in her brassiere to increase the size; and my sister and I had written signs to keep her out of trouble. But I didn't want my mother to give up another inch. I didn't want to stop being her child.

Old friends (or so I thought them) continued telling Margaret and me things about Allene, hinting at things about her — that she had never "lived all that well, if you know what I mean, dear." No, I didn't. And it wasn't important. She had done a really good job with us, I thought. She had made me react with disdain at hearing back-room gossip, and that's good, I thought. I heard things about fights that broke up friendships of half a lifetime; I heard she was a great flirt, but I knew that; I heard she'd had affairs; and I heard that some people never liked her; and one woman actually had the nerve to tell my sister that Allene had "gotten what she deserved." I didn't happen to think so. I remembered my mother as that woman teaching those children, that beauty on the other end of the ski rope, that woman who got me out of bed every day and encouraged me to fight back, that graceful woman who was loved by that wonderful man who was never wrong. I heard a lot. I knew a great deal, and at the time I decided that I didn't want to know any more.

But I did.

Chapter 13

"My name is Marion Roach. I am one of two daughters of a victim of Alzheimer's disease."

I was looking Claude Pepper in the eye and testifying in Congress before the House Subcommittee on Aging. At my right sat a man whose father was just acquitted after pumping a fatal shot into his wife, who was an Alzheimer's victim. To the right of the table were television cameras and radio and TV newspeople. It was August 1983.

"Late in 1979 I began to think that my mother was going mad. I called it madness — to myself — at first, because I found her behavior impossible to understand or explain.

"My mother was an independent and willful person. In her life she has been a precious only child, a good student, a beautiful sorority sister, a newspaper reporter, a wife, a mother, a Girl Scout leader, a Visiting Nurse volunteer, and a teacher at a bilingual preschool on the Lower East Side of Manhattan.

"In the progression of her disease she had been forgetful, then frightened, depressed, angry, paranoid, hostile, and incompetent. She is now completely dependent upon the aid of others. She cannot be left alone. She is repetitive and confused. She is agitated. She cannot read. She cannot drive. She cannot always form complete sentences. She frequently speaks rapid gibberish. She cannot bathe properly. She has no short-term memory. With the progression of her disease, she will almost assuredly lose control over all of her bodily functions; she will have to be fed, bathed, and dressed. My mother is fifty-four years old."

I looked up. I had made enough of these speeches that summer to know where it was that people got their feelings hurt. People always winced when they heard her age. They should have.

"She is suffering from senility. She is suffering from the humiliation of having her dignity wrenched from her. She is losing her mind in handfuls."

My testimony took twenty minutes. I saw myself on the news that night and I was glad that I looked so angry. I hadn't realized it while testifying, but I was mad. I was damn mad. And I had vented my anger in the best possible arena. I wanted someone to listen, and I had been as graphic and as angry as I could be, because I wanted to make them cry and I wanted them to change their laws and help us.

By the time of that testimony, my energy had become something of a fury. I had testified the previous week before a New York State Assembly hearing on Alzheimer's disease. I was working with Mayor Edward Koch and the New York City Department for the Aging on bringing together all the health, welfare, and service-related agencies in the city for a mayoral conference on Alzheimer's disease. I had spoken at nursing homes and at conferences. I had been on six talk shows, and I had reached the point where I could look Representative Pepper in the eye and tell him that my mother was losing her mind in handfuls, because she was, and that the federal insurance system stank, because it did. And still does.

All of a sudden the disease was chic. The year before, the month of November was made Alzheimer's month, but no one had paid a great deal of attention. Now we had a mayoral conference set to kick off the month in New York, New York State Senate hearings coming up, and speeches throughout the month. There were books coming out and appearances being made by doctors, lawyers I knew, people I had worked with.

It was very exciting. But there were irresponsible items in the press — reports of wonder drugs, reports that aluminum was the cause.

It is true that in the brains of some Alzheimer's victims large amounts of aluminum are found at autopsy. But it is also true that in states where alum is not used to purify the water (the main source of our intake of aluminum) there is no aluminum found in the brains of the Alzheimer's victims.

I remembered when I first heard about aluminum. I stopped using anything in cans, threw out cookware. And it was happening again. More and more reports were showing up in the press about the research on aluminum, and more people were reacting somewhat hysterically.

But the publicity helped. People were talking about the disease. Money, though in small amounts, was trickling in more steadily.

I went to visit my mother one Saturday at the end of the summer. We had lunch. She loves to eat, and usually we stay in when I visit, but I decided we'd go out — which meant a diner now, not the club. Why do all women in Queens with long nails and balding husbands go to diners on beautiful Saturday afternoons?

We have to go to diners. Those people don't. We have to go because my mother is so agitated that she leaps up and hurls herself into a bathroom every several minutes whether at home or in public.

In a restaurant, there is no seating right next to the bathroom. In a diner, there is. Even with this problem, it's worth it, because she's gotten out of the house; it's worth it to see her smile.

The place was packed, and managing to get a seat next to the bathroom was difficult. It was the second diner we had tried. We had had to leave the first place five minutes after arriving because we were too far from the bathroom and my mother went into a visible panic.

The scene was a movie, if anyone was watching. There we sat, in our second cavernous diner of the day, this one with tufted silver upholstery, I holding my mother's arm to the table — to keep her there for a moment, anyway — and the waitress standing over us waiting for our order. The waitress was actually snapping her gum.

The menu was enormous and laminated. The first heading in the first wide column was headed, "Meat Sandwiches."

My mother looked up at the waitress, said, "Meat sandwich," closed her menu, leaped up from the table, and dashed for the bathroom. While she was away I ordered a Reuben sandwich for her. I remember the first time I had one. She had ordered it in a restaurant and I thought it was neat. No ham on white for her. Something different, just like her.

In our fifty-five-minute lunch she went to the bathroom eleven times. And that was when I couldn't stop her. Mostly, she didn't do much in a bathroom. Most of the time she just stood facing the toilet for a moment, stared at it, and then pushed the plunger with her foot.

She glared at her Reuben sandwich when it finally came. She touched it with a finger, pushed it to the end of the platter. Then she stopped and shoved her long nails into her pleated paper cup of cole slaw.

I suggested a knife and fork.

"Knife and fork?" she asked, quietly.

I handed hers to her. She turned the utensils in one hand and put them down and went back to the cole slaw with her fingers. I handed the knife and fork back to her, and she used them, gingerly and suspiciously. At one point I was holding one of her arms down on the table while she ate with the other hand, with a fork, the whole time her half-chewed Reuben sandwich tumbling from her mouth, while she sputtered, "I have to go to the bathroom. Marion, I really have to go."

"Two more bites, please, then go."

"Okay."

Across the way a mother was leaning down to a child, saying, "One piece at a time, please."

We were speaking the same language. But I had tears in my eyes.

"Well, it's nice to see you," my mother said, breaking my sad concentration. "I like being here. It's nice to see you."

It made my day.

"You too, Ma, really."

"Marion, I have to go to the bathroom."

And she tore away from the table.

I sat there, thinking about our last visit to Dr. Reisberg, two weeks before this lunch. I had driven out from the city, picked her up, driven her in for the exam, out again, and then back to the city, after which I lay on my bed and cried for the first time in weeks. A long, hard cry. I had changed my hope. Now I hoped we would survive, my sister and I.

After the examination, when my mother was in the bathroom, Dr. Reisberg said to me, "Well, you should be happy. There doesn't seem to be any deterioration from six months ago and very little from a year ago. She could stay at this stage for three years."

My hope was different, Doctor. Couldn't you see?

Apparently, he could see. "What's wrong, Marion? You look . . ."

I was wrenched out of my thoughts by a hand on my back. It was my mother, standing over me in the diner.

"Marion," she said, "I really miss your father."

"Me too." I looked at my plate. I missed him desperately, yet I was glad that he'd never seen this.

She sat down again. "When can I come back to the house?" she asked, reaching across and touching my arm. But before I could answer, she asked, "Why am I living in an apartment?"

"Because the roof fell in."

On the way home from the diner we listened to a Billie Holiday tape. My mother kept snapping her fingers and talking about the music. She would speak some of the lyrics, repeating them, after the song had gone on to another line, as if she were savoring them. After I dropped her off at her apartment, I sat in the car and thought more about that last examination with Dr. Reisberg, about his saying that I should be happy.

He had started the examination by asking, "Mrs. Roach, what did you do this summer?"

"May I have a cup of coffee? May I smoke?" she answered.

It was her fourth cigarette in thirty minutes, the fifth time she had asked for coffee, which she was not allowed to drink. The caffeine made her more agitated. She had been getting up at two-thirty in the morning, every morning, and sitting by the front door. It was driving her attendants crazy. No one was getting any sleep. That was why we had come to Dr. Reisberg, so that he could increase the medication to keep her sedated through the night.

My mother could not get out the front door of the apartment alone. She tried, though, over and over. There was a large slab of a lock on the inside, and the attendant slept with the key. My mother had been sitting up every night, sitting and smoking, waiting for dawn.

"No, Ma, no coffee, no caffeine, remember?" Why did I still say "remember"?

"Mrs. Roach, what did you do this summer?" Dr. Reisberg repeated.

"May I smoke?"

She had a lit cigarette in front of her.

"Mrs. Roach, you like sports, is that right?"

"Yes."

"Did you do any sports this summer?"

"May I have a cup of coffee?"

"Mrs. Roach, did you go sailing this summer?"

"I lost my Nimblet in the hurricane of 1936. Ernie Bilhuber didn't tie it right."

It came out as a slur. "Boat" was a buzz word that always elicited this response, word for word, but rushed. "Sailing" was a buzz word. "Hurricane," too. Each got the same response. It was one of the six stories she told. If you said, "tulips," she'd tell you when she was born. "Boat," and she'd tell you about her Nimblet. When she looked at me, she knew I was someone she loved, but she wasn't sure which one.

Dr. Reisberg looked at me, puzzled by the jammed response about the Nimblet. I said it slowly for him. I knew it by heart. I hated repeating it.

"But did you go sailing this summer?" he asked again.

"My daughter took me sailing and I played tennis and I swam."

"Oh, I see," Dr. Reisberg said.

"Is this correct?" he asked me, the traitor, the daughter-spy.

"No, no."

I was getting better at this. I didn't cry. I hardly looked

out the window these days. I used to get stomachaches. Then, for a while, I wanted to kill her. Now I wanted to change the channel. But I didn't cry.

"No, she hasn't been sailing this summer."

My mother looked at me. She was angry. Then her anger turned to confusion, a shred of self-defense.

"May I have a cup of coffee?" she asked.

I had not taken my mother sailing since August 1982, the year before. She was large and clumsy. She forgot what she ate and therefore ate continuously. If there were six yogurts in the refrigerator, they would have been gone in three hours; a carton of ice cream, a gallon of soda. She ate anyone's food. She gained twenty pounds in a few months. She had no balance.

The last time she'd been sailing she teetered around Skip's forty-seven-foot boat. She could not sit still, and as the thirty-foot boom swung over her head, I kept imagining her standing up at the wrong moment and being thrown over the side. The only thing that kept her in her place was the tape player — one of those briefcases of music. I had come prepared with Ella Fitzgerald, Billie Holiday, and Frank Sinatra. She sat and listened, flipping the pages of her appointment book. Between songs she would look up and ask whoever was closest, "What day is it?" "When do I play tennis?" "Is this Wednesday?" When she did get up, she knocked things over and left cigarettes burning throughout the boat.

We were sitting calmly, having run out of wind and turned on the engine. We were all sitting there when we smelled smoke. It was in the engine compartment. Skip thought that it might be an electrical fire and in an instant dived below decks and started directing me to put everyone into life jackets and over the side.

I went below, after him. It was a wooden boat; it could have gone up in an instant. Skip was an excellent sailor and a very careful man. I trusted his sailing ability completely. Now, I looked at him and stopped.

"What are you doing?" he asked me, somewhat hysterically. "Go on, get them over the side."

"You want me to put her over the side?" I shrieked. All I could envision was my mother floating down Long Island Sound, reading her date book. "You want me to watch her bob up and down around out there asking what day it is and what time it is and do you really think I am going to do that?" I screamed, grabbing him by his shoulders, shaking him.

He looked at me, shut his eyes for an instant, and snorted. He wrenched the fire extinguisher from its metal clasps and covered the engine compartment, the aftercabin, himself, and me in foam. No one went over the side, but he took a terrible risk.

"What else did you do this summer, Mrs. Roach," asked Dr. Reisberg.

"I played tennis every day."

"Is this true?" to me.

"No."

She rarely played tennis. The people at the club shunned her. Lette pursued it, taking her, defending her, tearing into the women who were unkind, thanking the ones who were patient, but it was getting to be too much. Lette wouldn't admit it, but we knew.

I wondered how many of those people who were mean deserved my understanding. I understood that it was difficult for them. But it was difficult for Allene. She was lonely and scared and quiet. And she was senile. They could not imagine the terror that was whipping through her mind. She was much less aware of her illness than she was three years ago, but she still knew, and it embarrassed her.

"Do you still swim, Mrs. Roach? I remember that you used to swim."

She looked at me. God, I felt like such a traitor. She was looking at me with anger and with fear, daring me to answer but afraid that her own answer would be wrong.

"Sometimes."

Good girl, Ma. When in doubt, wing it. That's my mom.

Actually, she had become terrified of the water. The terror is common to her disease. At home, every morning in her apartment, she would put on her shower cap, clench her jaw, relax it, clench it again, sliding her upper teeth over her lower, and stand outside the shower, staring at the water. Clenching and relaxing. Clenching.

The daughter of another victim told me that her mother recently started shrieking when she saw a full bathtub. She told her daughter that she was afraid of going down the drain.

The next week I was sitting at my Wednesday night Alzheimer's support group meeting. Roberta had just returned from her honeymoon in Italy. She and Peter had taken leave from their separate jobs defending the law, and they both looked terrific and rested and decked out in the latest Italian fashion. Life went on. Roberta and I had become good friends, and I cherished that. Because of these meetings, this disease, we were friends. And in spite of it.

I was talking about what gave my mother joy.

She wasn't much of a person. What I meant was that there wasn't much of a person's whole life left that she could exhibit. She was not conversational. She didn't like to talk. She could walk and she could eat. And she could smile.

My mother loved her music. She remembered all the words to "Witchcraft," "Moonglow," "September Song," and every other song I could find on tape. She smiled, and we sat through one side and she'd just play it all again if I didn't flip it over for her. She liked to listen to the music. Something inside her made her just glow with the songs. She was slightly ungainly in her step, but on the couch, hands folded, Frank Sinatra in the background, she was happy, and that made me happy, too. I liked to talk about it. Knowing that something made her happy made me glad she was alive.

There were two new people in the group. New people brought the worst heartaches, because they were hopeful and because as they heard us speak about how to wash a victim, how to brush their teeth, we could almost hear the hope seep from them.

A woman who had been in the group for several years was talking about her son, George, who was going to apply to college in the spring. Marta's husband had not recognized his son since the boy was twelve. The father, once a famous engineer, had been in a nursing home with Alzheimer's disease for two years.

Marta had gone to the home the day before to find another dementia patient holding his hand. A woman. The woman asked Marta if the male attendant was "her man." She asked if the husband was her father.

Marta said, "No, this is my man," pointing to her husband, who hadn't recognized her the day before.

The woman tossed his hand at his chest and said, "You didn't tell me you were married."

We all laughed. Marta laughed. And then she looked at the table. "When I looked at my husband, there were two thick tears running down his cheeks. He recognized me that day."

She went on to tell about George and his plans for college. He had been asked to write an essay about the person he most wanted to meet. He had been thinking about it for weeks and the day before came to his mother with his decision.

"He is going to write about his father," she said, proudly. "Everyone tells him how talented his father was. He never knew this. He was too young when his father got sick. Everyone tells him how good his work was, how much good he did. George said, 'I want to meet that man.' "

Three times when I was a child, my mother dragged me out of bed in the middle of the night to watch a movie. The first was *From Here to Eternity*. My mother told me that it was the story of a comeback. I didn't see any comeback, I said afterward, rubbing my eyes at dawn.

"Frank Sinatra," she said, not sleepy. "This is where Frank Sinatra made his comeback. It is possible."

I was confused. She had always told me that there are no comebacks, no patch-ups; that when something was leaking, it was sinking.

The next movie was *A Streetcar Named Desire*. Again, I was sleepy and confused.

"Men," she said. "This one is about the type of man all women find attractive."

In an undershirt?

The third movie was *A Night to Remember*, about the sinking of the *Titanic*. "I would have gotten on one of those lifeboats," she said. "You have to do that," she said. "You have to do what you must to survive."

To survive my mother's illness, I finally knew that I had to separate myself from her. I would never give her up, but I had to cut the connection, which was pulling me down with her. I had to separate the illness from her. The woman she had been would never leave me, but the body that housed this maniacal disease would, and I had to survive. She had told me that.

But Margaret and I had to ensure her survival. There is a fine line between managing a person well and teaching a person helplessness. It is difficult in the beginning to sit through the task that the victim is struggling with — fumbling with her keys, staring at the buttons on a sweater, forgetting to lick envelopes. It is even more difficult to know when to take over, when to unlock the door.

The desire, in the beginning, is to allow the shower to take longer, to be possibly less than perfect in its execution, in order to prolong independence and self-respect for both the victim and the viewer. But as the disease progresses, the act becomes more complicated.

When do you go in the bathroom and watch? When do you get in the shower and help? When do you get in the shower and administer the entire act? Do you ever, if you are the child of the victim? The spouse? Is that an act, a humiliation, better performed by a hired person, a non-relative? Does the mother become a patient, an object to be bathed instead of a mother, when the child is in the shower, soaping the washcloth, lifting her arms?

We had no rule of thumb. We had no guidebook. My sister and I believed that the first and most important aspect of our mother's care was to preserve what remained of her awareness, to keep her in a social environment as long as possible, outside an institution.

To do this we developed a small network of helpers. There were several friends of my mother who still visited and continued to provide activities.

And there was Pat.

Pat was a member of the local Catholic church. She visited my mother for the bulk of the day, four days each week. She took Allene bowling and to one of those exercise places, to the movies and shopping. My mother loved Pat. They were friends. They drove around the neighborhood and they smoked cigarettes together and Pat cared.

Early in the relationship between Allene and Pat, some of the women at my mother's tennis club were very mean to Pat. One took her aside and suggested that "those girls" must be paying her a great deal to take care of such "an animal." My mother. This from someone who had lived in the community nearly as long as my mother. This from a contemporary of my mother with children. An animal? Because she was confused? This at a stage when Allene was still playing tennis but wasn't sure how to score. This before the ugliest phases. My mother, an animal?

We didn't hear this from Pat. She never would have repeated something someone had said to her. She never would, even in a quote, call my mother an animal. It was weeks after the incident, after Pat had asked us not to pay her anymore, had said that she wanted to come without charge (the pay was minimal at best). Another woman told Margaret, and through Lette we made known our horror, but the criticism continued. Pat attended the same church as most of the people in the community. She was one of the kindest, strongest, most quietly loyal people I have ever met, and they were criticizing her clothes and her attentive care of my mother.

In the beginning I thought such behavior was the consequence of people being afraid of this disability: the fear bred panic — cruelty through fear. But I don't know. That part about "animal" is unforgivable.

At the apartment, most of the seven-day week was first covered by Flo. Flo was a piece of work. You'd have thought the place was the chummiest sorority house — and the cleanest — going. Flo and my mother watched television and wore matching sweaters. They kissed each other and held hands. Flo would kiss Allene goodbye and vice versa. Flo was not afraid to touch, and my mother began to respond, after a short time, to the tenderness of Flo, after all those years of saying that touching was silly. My mother began to respond to an arm on her arm, a hug from her family, and it was Flo who taught us not to be afraid to give it. It was a very effective way of getting and keeping Allene's attention.

Her memory was so bad that when I sat with her and she looked out the window and then looked back at me, she would say, "Oh, how are you?" as though I had just entered the room. It could go on like that all day, with the conversation never getting any further, unless I sat next to her with my hand on her arm or holding her hand. Then, her attention was on me. But we had never been like that, and it was Flo who taught me that this new person liked to be touched.

I think some people fear this disease is contagious. Flo didn't. Neither did Pat.

Because of the various women who stayed with Allene — and there were dozens, from agencies, from local organizations, from friends — there was a shifting of decisions that left the day-to-day care — the dressing, the bathing, the feeding — of Allene in the hands of others. We came around a painful circle and in the process picked up some new family, but we also lost a piece of a fight. We couldn't do it alone.

What began with Eva, our housekeeper, our friend, was inherited by women from agencies. We thought that someone who didn't know us too well would give more professional care and have less personal involvement, less grief, than someone like Eva, who loved my mother very much.

A whole world opened up to us then: phone calls with advice from the people as they got to know Margaret better, complaints about the weekend person who ate all the chicken, the weekend person who said there was nothing to eat. We didn't expect that — or the uniforms.

At first, this was a real issue. Neither Margaret nor I wanted uniforms sitting there, in church with my mother, in the kitchen, greeting my mother every morning, reminding her that she was sick. We held the line for a long time. But people seem to like uniforms, and every time I would just drop by, every time Margaret made one of her frequent but unannounced visits, there would be a white ribbed dress, and we finally just gave in. The uniform separates the ill from the sick, the healer from the victim. I guess to some it is a way of keeping their distance. To others, it is the mark of a professional. I had to learn to take these reasons into consideration and to respect the wishes of others. But I never got accustomed to them.

Through every aspect of my mother's illness, we greeted the new wrinkle, we fought it, we relinquished some control. It was a Depression dance marathon that no one ever wins.

One day I was on the phone with my mother and then with Flo. Flo asked whether I had "sent the money."

Leading with my chin, as always, I asked, "What money?"

"The money."

I figured that if it was a small sum, I could certainly get Skip or Scott to drop off a couple of dollars. Margaret was at work and I was in Manhattan.

"How much do you need?" I asked.

"Oh, quite a bit."

"Uh, Flo, what for?"

"I want to take your mother on a little trip."

"What?"

"A trip. A little trip. I just want the money for the bus fare. I'll pay the rest."

"Where?"

"Atlantic City."

"What?" I had heard it, but, well, come on.

"Atlantic City. You know, New Jersey?"

"Why?"

"To play the machines."

I told Flo I would have to call her back. I got into bed and put the covers over my head and stayed there for an hour. Then I called back and talked her out of the idea. I could picture it all too well, Flo with one arm locked onto my mother and the other pulling the handle. I didn't think it was a good idea. I didn't think, before that day, that I would ever have to confront such ideas. We never knew what was next, and that's why there was no rule of thumb. You can't live each day as if it were your last. You just live it, and the next day you laugh when you see an advertisement for Atlantic City.

My mother continued to change every day. We would sit in her apartment and she would stare at the television. She listened to her tapes. I would chatter on about my day, her apartment, Margaret's garden, hoping that my mother would jump in and participate, and occasionally she would. But then the feedback dwindled to nothing.

I used to think that without it there was no communication, and without communication there was no relationship. I used to think that without current conversation, the everyday exchanges, there was no future for a relationship. I was wrong.

Not even death can alter imitation. It can't steal her favorite phrases from us, her gestures, her ferocious curiosity, her romantic notions. They are in me and they are in Margaret, although they are different — so very different — in each of us.

Sometimes you have only to walk like someone to have that person there with you. Sometimes you have only to wear a hat or mismatch your socks. We feel and act the way we do, my sister and I, because of the way we feel about Allene. It can be altered, and that's good, but it cannot be taken away.

Chapter 14

ASLEEP. I had had a long, aromatic Indian dinner earlier with Dr. Reisberg. We were both to speak at a conference the following week and were comparing notes.

I am in my apartment on the West Side alone, happy, and asleep.

Asleep with the windows open. It is 1:40 in the morning. Asleep under the salmon-pink satin comforter that was Marion Rollins Zillmann's and under the quilt that was made in 1930. The date is embroidered on the corner in lavender. It was made by another ancestor.

Asleep and warm, and the breeze is soft and cool. I stretch over the brass bed and pick up the ringing phone, which is on the floor.

"I used to tell the most beautiful stories to children. To Eddie's children. He has two, and another on the way. The stories were beautiful and long. They were easy to tell. I do not do it anymore. You have to help me. I need to tell them again. You must come to me and help me."

"It's you," I said, and I smiled, thinking about the King of Scotland.

"Are you smiling?"

"I am," I said, smiling in the dark. "Where are you?"

"I am here and you must come to me. I am in Boston. Get on a plane in the morning. We are going to the country. Is your hair long?"

"Yes. Do you have any left?"

"Bitch. Come to me and everything will be different."

"I will."

"I will call you in the morning. Get a plane schedule. Get here as early as you can. I need to tell stories to children."

I decide to take the eleven o'clock shuttle to Boston.

It is two in the morning. I am lying in the breeze and I cannot help marveling at the magic of the call, the words. I cannot help thinking that this time, like the last, he has appeared just when I need him.

The phone rings. "Are you still smiling?"

"Yes. I'll be there at twelve."

"I'll be at the airport."

It's been five and a half years since we last saw each other, when my father died; more than eight years since we first met, when I was on my way to London and Africa. Years and years of believing that there could be such a man, and then these eight years of knowing that there is — years, after meeting him, of dreaming he'd come back, as my mother liked to say to get me, "if you play your cards right." But in the last five and a half years so many things have changed — except this dream.

I have lost weight. I have new clothes, the outfits of a young adult woman. I am on the plane and I am reading. I am trying to contain my nerves, trying to pretend that I don't want it to be just like a remake of the movie *Gigi* or like all those lyrics in all those songs my mother loved and from which, I realize, I have taken most of my notions of romance.

It is a beautiful, cool day. In the airport there are tourists, and I am carrying my bag. I didn't know how much to bring, because he wouldn't tell me how long he'd be here.

I am wearing an Italian suit I bought a few months before. "Ah, you. Look at you," he says with that Scottish lilt, a voice of a gray suede glove, sliding down a banister.

I just press my palm into his, which is upturned, and offer my cheek, longing to be elegant and controlled, but secretly dying to jump up and down. It's too incredible that it's he, here, now.

In another minute I am sloped in the back seat of a long limousine in Boston, and he is strangely better-looking, even without the fur coat.

Eddie is with him, and we are going to Lexington and Concord to see the bridge where the shot heard round the world was fired. There is chilled champagne, which we sip while the buildings of Boston turn into the leaves of early autumn in the small towns. We stop at an inn and have lunch and we tease about our looks and I say that he has more hair than he did and he changes the subject.

"Look how you've grown up. Are you trying to be a greyhound? You are so long and tall and thin. My God, Eddie, I never thought that kid in the T-shirts would grow up. Where is that baby fat, child?"

"The same place some of your hair is, my vain darling; moved around," I say, realizing that he has transplanted some of his hair to the top.

"Ah. Maybe she's not all grown up yet, Eddie. Tell me, how is your mother, your sister?"

I had sent him a copy of the magazine piece and had never gotten a response. But then he almost never wrote. And we never called.

"Didn't you get the magazine?"

"Yes, it was good, but I didn't know the *New York Times Magazine* published fiction. Tell me, why did you wish me here? I have had the most powerful feelings about you recently. That's why I decided to come and see you. What's this all about?"

This stuff is supposed to happen only in romance novels, I think, but he's here and this is the way he talks and I had been wishing for him, but I had not received a word until the call from Boston.

"Hm," I replied, just wondering if this was all going to come out as I had hoped, "that story was real."

"No."

"Didn't you get my letter?"

"No letter. It can't be real. When did I see her? Five years ago, when I was in New York. Oh, God, but she was so beautiful. She's young."

Later, lying down, clutching. "What is it, child? Why do you need to be held like this?"

"Because it is true and because it is not what I expected. Ever."

God, I hoped I was playing my cards right. I hoped I wasn't scaring him away.

There is a type of confidence that can be taught, and I was the perfect student. When he was first teaching his sales group in South Africa to sell, he would drive them around in a van. If it was raining, he would never use the wipers. He would drive up and pick up his crew and he would leave the wipers off. He would not let them know that he acknowledged the weather.

His staff never say *if*. They carry whistles, and when anyone says *if*, they all blow them. "Never say if; say when. Never say cold. It is never cold. It is fresh," he told me, sitting there in the vast hotel lobby in Boston.

He got up to speak with the desk clerk. Within three minutes there were four clerks, leaning over the counter, enchanted.

"Can't means won't, so say it if you won't, but do anything if you can," he said to them. One of them had told him that they "can't" find the name of a restaurant he wanted.

He had a black cape with a brocade collar clasp and a

silver lining, "like every cloud." And he had a small splash of lines next to his eyes.

We went to the oldest restaurant in the city, where there were silver tray covers that had chains running to the ceiling in a dark wooden room. We danced to the music we hummed, twirling through the downstairs in the room with the covers when there was no one there. It was late, and we had been ordering California wines. The next day we shopped along the streets of Boston and bought tapes he couldn't get in South Africa.

Back at the hotel, he saw his first video on the cable television and sat, like a child, with his legs crossed and his palms to his chin, and I could see him planning.

That night he wrapped me in that cape and we went out and had champagne in a lively club. He said we were "putting on the ritz."

The next day we went to the river and had lobsters for lunch. We each had one, and then, still hungry, we each had another. Neither one of us would wear the paper bibs. The waiter introduced himself by first name, the way they do these days.

"I am Douglas, the King of Scotland," said he in return, "and this is a young woman who used to be a child and sometimes still is."

The waiter asked me what I wanted.

"Boxing gloves."

The poor waiter. He never had a chance. We practically upended the table, sloshing through the butter, cracking claws, ordering more, and bantering, grabbing, and kissing.

We had a walk along the water and I told him about all that had happened with my mother, starting right after my father's death.

"Were you scared?" he asked, lifting my chin, looking into my eyes.

"No."

"Remember that, then. Don't be, don't ever be. Except of me." The big bad wolf.

We came back from another shopping spree up and down Newbury Street. He was looking at fabrics, comparing them with the big red bow he had gotten to put around the Rolls-Royce he had bought his mother and was on his way to deliver to her before returning to South Africa. When we got back to the room he got a glass of water and popped something into his mouth. I asked him what it was.

"A browning pill," he replied.

"Hm?"

"It makes you brown. Tan, I think you say. I have been on vacation for three weeks and mostly I have worked, but I don't want anyone to know that when I get back. I want them to think I've been at the beach. And when I get home it will be summer and I want to be tan."

"What's in them, the pills?"

I was trying on the cape again, clasping the collar.

"I don't know."

"What the hell do you mean, you don't know? They could be poison; probably are. Tanning. What a lot of nonsense. They could kill you, for God's sake. What are you, crazy? You want to die by the time you're fifty-five?"

He was thirty-six, I finally managed to find out. Fifty-five stuck in my head. It seemed awfully young to be terribly ill.

"I'm not going to live that long," he said.

"What the hell are you saying? Don't talk nonsense. You of all people must want to live that long."

Thirty-six and he's living as though he just wants to be a good-looking corpse — living as though he doesn't want to live very long.

"No, no I don't," he went on, "and I won't. Not the way I live. I want to enjoy my life. I just want to live each day as if it were my last."

Not I.

Chapter 15

I AM NOT living today as if it were my last. People get hurt that way. But I am not living today, as those silly posters suggest, as if it were the first day, either.

I neglected to return my "no book this month" card to my book club, so the mailman brought a book I did not order. It was about managing stress. I had to laugh. I opened it. The book directed the reader to develop a strategy for living with stress. It told the reader that the best-managed stress is stress that one can see coming, can prepare for.

I rarely think that way.

Recently Margaret said to me, with some exasperation, "I never know what's going to happen next."

I replied, "Thank God." Good or bad, I don't want to know.

The book was correct: having the right attitude helps. But I — simple and stubborn — will always wish my mother had never gotten sick. Before I react I always say to myself that I wish she weren't sick. Always. Then I react. I am not resigned to it, and therefore I react the way I do. I don't assess it very well. I never ask why. I just wish it weren't so, and then do what I think is right. But I always make that wish first.

How I take her illness is up to me, but long before she

became sick she got me to love her to this degree and taught me to believe with all my heart the things in which I believe. It's nice that someone wants me to manage my stress. But instead of a handbook about what to do with the wreckage, I prefer to remember that, under every and all stress, the best prevention against self-destruction is love.

Live each day as if it were my last. No thanks. My mother was wrong about that. She was wrong about a lot of other things, too, but that doesn't make me love her any less. She was wrong, or I was wrong, or we were both wrong, about romance and love. Many people liked to tell me that she had had an affair. All I know is what I've heard, but more important, I don't care about it. Romance, the way I wanted it, the way I learned it in the lyrics she and I loved, is grand and fun, and I wouldn't trade the chance I had at nineteen to have a grand romance, though I was wrong to think it was love.

But she was right when she taught me to accept when I am wrong or when something is over, and to allow myself to change and adjust and not just cling to it out of habit. When it's over, it's over, she said.

My mother's illness made a huge lunge at her mind in the fall of 1983, and after that, abilities slid from her without a struggle. Even the slightest inklings would extinguish themselves as quickly as tiny firecrackers directed right into a pond; I'd see a flicker, and then nothing.

Margaret and I went to her apartment on Christmas morning. Our mother sat staring at the packages in her lap. We opened them for her; the new shirt, the nightgown, received the same fixed look of nonrecognition.

In January of 1984, I was on my way to dinner, on a snowy night, when Margaret called, sounding very hesitant. She was choosing her words carefully; then she blurted out that Allene had become incontinent. There had been little accidents, apparently, that Pat had witnessed, but all of a sudden it began to happen, in the apartment, according to Flo, during the day and every night. I was supposed to be outside waiting for a friend to pick me up in a cab; my buzzer rang and I got off the phone. I went through dinner with a smile slapped onto my face, came home, lit a fire in the fireplace, and cried into my palms. It was days before I spoke to anyone about it. I could not stand the idea of my mother enduring the embarrassment of incontinence.

We gained and lost help. Flo, who had been so wonderful, reached a state of exhaustion common to those doing her kind of work. She was replaced by Ivy, who was equally wonderful. Ivy, like Flo, worked Monday through Friday, twenty-four hours each day. But the weekend people came and went so fast that I had to ask their names each time I called.

Over and over Margaret or I would introduce a new person to Allene. "Her name is Allene. She likes to be called by her first name. She is very confused. She will eat if you place the food in front of her and continue to remind her to eat. She doesn't sleep well during the night. She will get up often. She's not violent. She's very sweet, aren't you, Mommy?"

She and I would be sitting on the couch, a new companion, in uniform, sitting across the room. My mother wouldn't even nod. "She's very sweet. She was very smart," I'd say, gripping Allene's hand. I would have tears in my eyes, and I'd be hoping this stranger would care enough about my mother not to be harsh with her. I wanted Allene to be liked and understood. But all we were paying them for was to keep her clean, fed, and dressed.

Early in the spring, while visiting, I saw the lock on the door.

On the outside of my mother's bedroom there was a hook-and-eye lock. It meant that she was being locked in at night.

I spoke about it with Ivy. She and Margaret had agreed that it was the thing to do. My mother was getting up every night and trying to get out of the apartment. The kitchen door was locked; the door to the patio was locked; the windows were locked. She couldn't go anywhere, but she would try, and no one was getting any sleep. She was locked in her room, and I imagined her pacing in there, not understanding why she couldn't get out, just pacing. Then I realized that if the companions were getting sleep, they were doing a better job and they were happier and my mother was getting better care. And I knew that she'd get out of bed, go to the door, try it, go back to bed, get out again, walk to the door, return to bed . . . Putting on the lock was the right thing to do.

The money was going very fast. We were trying to find a roommate for Allene, another Alzheimer's victim, but were having a hard time. We wanted someone at her stage of the illness. The costs were, as Peter Strauss had predicted, $4000 a month, and we were nearing the end of my mother's savings in the trust. It hadn't been even a year, and we were racing this demon. Which was going to happen first? A roommate? Allene's going into a home? Her death? Every day was another question of management. Margaret was being barraged with phone calls from the companions about what to feed Allene and when to feed her, about daily activities. The super wanted to know why the weekend people kept changing all the time and why none of them ever did the right thing with the garbage. The calls were constant.

In March Mayor Edward Koch of New York officially announced the opening of an Alzheimer's office for information and referral. The commissioner of the Department for the Aging, Janet Sainer, appointed Randi Goldstein to head it, and I was very pleased. Now there were two places in the city to get help: our New York chapter of the Alzheimer's Disease and Related Disorders Association and this new office. There was help available.

By April, Allene was almost totally housebound. She fretted so badly when she was away from a bathroom that a walk became only an exercise in agitation. She had two subjects on which she could form complete sentences: the bathroom and wanting a cigarette.

And by April both Margaret and I had started in therapy. We would talk about it on the phone. We talked about Allene and our different feelings about her, and sometimes, it turned out, we had talked about the very same things in the same week at our separate sessions. She was going to a therapist on Long Island; I was going to a therapist in Manhattan. The sessions were a great help for me. I had thought that all my private fears and problems were related to my mother's illness; I had blamed every fault of mine on my grief. And I was terribly wrong.

In May I received a call from a man who ran a nursing home in Riverdale. I had made a speech there the year before and at the time had promised to come back and have a tour. We had run into each other at a meeting of the board in the mayoral office on which we both served, and he reminded me of my promise. I renewed it, though reluctantly. I was trying to be polite, and I figured he just wanted to show off his place.

Jacob Reingold is a remarkable man. He directs the Hebrew Home for the Aged, a huge and fascinating institution. The home was scheduled, within months, to begin construction of a wing devoted to care of Alzheimer's patients and research on the disease. We walked around the facility. It has a sloping lawn leading to the Hudson River. There are paintings and art exhibits. There is a cage of beautiful birds just off one of the dining rooms. There are eleven hundred residents. There is an apartment building for the healthy elderly who choose to live there; there is a museum on the grounds; there are movies and lectures and therapy programs. After the tour and lunch we went to his office. He asked me about my mother, and as I started to describe her, I began to cry.

He took my hands. He said, "Marion, you and your sister have done a wonderful job. You have your mother totally protected and cared for, but do you really think that after the nurses get finished bathing, feeding, and dressing your mother, they have time to talk with her, to stimulate her? You have created the perfect padded cell. It's time to see if she can be less helpless. Give a chance to those of us who know how to care for her. Put her in a home."

The words hung in the air. He was right: she had everything but stimulation. She was completely out of touch. She wasn't talking. She didn't seem happy; she seemed dead.

All that time I believed I was right, and now, in a minute, the objections to her being in a home lost all their strength. It hurt to think I had been wrong. It must have registered on my face.

"She has benefited from your care. Now she would benefit from being here. I promise you. I'm not trying to sell this home to you," he said. "I don't need the business, but you need my help."

Margaret and I discussed it. We were supporting her now. We started selling things. Margaret had a garage sale. We tried every measure to save money: buying food at the market farther from my mother's apartment, because it was cheaper; having Pat come fewer days. It was no use. We started selling my grandmother's silver, then jewelry. My mother never wore her wedding or engagement ring. Margaret asked me if I thought we should sell them. I said no. A few weeks later, I gave in.

Margaret gave me the name of a dealer downtown, a

friend of a friend. I cried all morning and then I went. The place was packed with little stalls of busy hands moving over cases of sold gems. I found the stall with the name of the woman my sister recommended and sat on the stool opposite the woman. I had brought handfuls of earrings and old gold necklaces of mine. I hadn't told my sister I was going to do this, but I thought it might help. I drew from my pocket the gold watch my parents had given me on my graduation from college, thrust it across the counter, and looked down, about to cry. There in the case was a necklace of Margaret's for which, I remember, she had saved for a year. Next to it, one of her rings, and next to that, costume jewelry of my mother's I remember using as dress-up when I was a child. I sold my mother's ring and left.

My mother entered the Fairfield Nursing Home in Riverdale at the end of August. It is owned by the Hebrew Home. It is smaller and provides the same delicate care. Everyone was very nice. I was very quiet. Grief is a mute sense of panic. I felt that I was letting go again, and I thought that perhaps I should panic and stop all this. But I knew better. I was quiet. It was the right thing to do.

On the door to room 308 was a sign in block letters. It read:

WELCOME Allene Roach to the Fairfield Nursing Home. We're happy you chose to live with us. We look forward to helping you participate in our daily activities.

We entered the room in which my mother was to live and saw the empty bed, with her name in a card holder above it. Margaret and I sat on opposite sides of the room and wept.

The anticipation of the experience was as far from the reality of the day as is, I hope, anticipating one's own death.

What I had dreaded most was saying goodbye and walking out of the room, leaving her there to live, leaving her there to die.

She didn't even notice when we left. She had a cookie in one hand and a cigarette in the other, and she was smiling at the nurse who had given her both. I kissed my mother on the side of her face and I left.

Within three months after my mother moved into the home, she regained what I estimated to be 20 percent of her speech. She was always with others — at music therapy, dance therapy, arts and crafts, current events class, and at meals. She recognized me now; three months ago she hadn't been quite sure who I was. She knew I was someone who loved her and someone whom she loved, but that was about it. At the home she'd ask me how I was. Not much more, but that was a lot.

She was fifty-six on Election Day of 1984. She knew it was her birthday. I brought her presents and some cookies, and she said to the nurse, looking at me, "That's my daughter. That's my kid."

My mother and I had been close friends. We went around together. One night right before the incident with the cats, we went to Carnegie Hall for a tribute to Hoagy Carmichael. He was there. The real reason that my mother wanted to go to the concert was that she had a crush on the bass player.

She had had a crush on him for a long time — for thirty years. He used to live in Douglaston. She said that he was the idol of her youth.

My mother looked terrific in bobby socks when she used to cut classes in high school to hear Frank Sinatra uptown. My father used to go to see the Marx Brothers for a nickel on Forty-second Street, and he saw Houdini. But my mother liked Frank Sinatra and this guy who played the bass.

We went to Carnegie Hall. She was supposed to meet me out front. I had paid for box tickets, because this was special. I loved Hoagy Carmichael. My mother had her bassist.

Actually they'd never really known each other too well. She had all his records, and she hummed the whistle section from "The Big Noise from Winnetka," whenever she thought no one was listening. She is tone deaf. Singing, she just swings at the key, any key, and misses. She always has. She joined a choir in Douglaston when she was a kid because her favorite boy was in it, and the choir director asked her to drop it. She's that tone deaf. They wouldn't just let her mouth the words.

The lights were dimming inside and she still wasn't there, in front, right between the two tall posters, as we'd planned. My mother was never late.

All of a sudden she came running around the corner. She was clutching her purse to her heart. She was smiling.

"Hey, Ma, I mean, you know, it's late. Where've you been?"

She looked at me with a question on her mind, as if I was supposed to know; as if I had neglected to wear my bobby socks for the first time; as if I had forgotten the rules.

"The stage door, as always," she said, skipping up the stairs. "Where were you?"

I'm right here, Allene.